Peter Brukner is a world-renowned sports and exercise medicine physician, researcher and public health advocate. Currently Professor of Sports Medicine at La Trobe University, Peter played an instrumental role in the development of sports medicine as a medical specialty in Australia, founded the largest multi-disciplinary sports medicine clinic in the country, and is the co-author of the most popular sports medicine textbook in the world, *Brukner & Khan's Clinical Sports Medicine*. Peter has also had team doctor roles with AFL, national swimming, hockey, athletics, soccer and cricket, as well as the Olympic Games, World Championships and Commonwealth Games. Peter was the Socceroos' team doctor at the 2010 World Cup, Head of Sports Medicine and Sports Science at Liverpool Football Club, and the Australian cricket team doctor from 2012–17.

As a consequence of his own personal health journey, Peter has become a passionate advocate of the importance of nutrition in the development of chronic diseases such as type 2 diabetes. He commenced the not-for-profit SugarByHalf in 2015 and published *A Fat Lot of Good* in 2019. In 2021 he launched Defeat Diabetes, the first Australian digital program to tackle the massive problem of type 2 diabetes.

Join the Defeat Diabetes movement:

Facebook: Defeat Diabetes Australia
Twitter: @defeatdiabetes_
Instagram: @defeatdiabetesau

T0274102

The Diabetes Plan

Dr Peter Brukner OAM

MACMILLAN
Pan Macmillan Australia

Pan Macmillan acknowledges the Traditional Custodians of country throughout Australia and their connections to lands, waters and communities. We pay our respect to Elders past and present and extend that respect to all Aboriginal and Torres Strait Islander peoples today. We honour more than sixty thousand years of storytelling, art and culture.

First published 2023 in Macmillan by Pan Macmillan Australia Pty Ltd
1 Market Street, Sydney, New South Wales, Australia, 2000

 A catalogue record for this book is available from the National Library of Australia

Typeset in 12.5/18 pt Sabon LT Pro by Post Pre-press Group

Printed by IVE

Internal photography by Defeat Diabetes, except Sesame Salmon Skewers, Super Simple Salmon Omelette, One-Pan Creamy Chicken and Mushroom, Cheesy Asparagus and Spinach Tart, and Quick Chicken Tikka Masala by istockphoto.

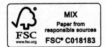 The paper in this book is FSC® certified. FSC® promotes environmentally responsible, socially beneficial and economically viable management of the world's forests.

With this book, I want to give HOPE to all those with type 2 diabetes and pre-diabetes – hope that you can reduce the impact of your condition and even put it into remission.

Contents

Foreword
by Dr James Muecke AM

Why should *you* 'defeat diabetes' with *The Diabetes Plan*?

Because you are likely one of the 14 million Australian adults who have insulin resistance, the driving force behind type 2 diabetes.

And what does type 2 diabetes look like?

Decades of unnecessary medical appointments, crippling expenses, lost work and life opportunities, and a battery of devastating complications: blindness, infertility, amputations, kidney failure, dementia, stroke, heart attack, untimely death . . . To name but a few.

Why should *we* 'defeat diabetes' with *The Diabetes Plan*?

Because type 2 diabetes is quite simply the biggest health crisis we have. Worldwide. 1.7 million cases in Australia. 28.9 million in the US. 65.9 million in India. 88.5 million in China. 537 million globally. And growing.

The cost to health systems and taxpayers is astronomical. And unsustainable.

The impact on our children is diabolical. And unforgiveable.

How can you defeat your own diabetes?

Type 2 diabetes is a disease of carbohydrate intolerance. Reducing your carbohydrate intake will go a long way towards improving your metabolic dysfunction. Perhaps even putting your type 2 diabetes into remission.

And for those in your family who are at risk, cutting back on sugar, refined carbs, 'vegetable' oils and ultra-processed consumables will likely prevent them from developing this insidious life-changing and life-threatening disease.

How can we defeat our diabetes epidemic?

Read Peter Brukner's timely and important book.

Share it with friends and family.

Share it with your GP and specialists.

Share it far and wide.

Type 2 diabetes should no longer be considered a progressive disease.

Medication, insulin and complications are not inevitable.

Although remission is not achievable for everyone,

it should be offered to everyone, and it should be attempted by everyone.

There is hope.

Together, let's work towards a world that is #type2free.

Together, let's defeat diabetes.

Dr James Muecke AM
Australian of the Year 2020

Introduction

When I was a medical student (a long time ago now!), I was told that:

'Type 2 diabetes is a chronic progressive disease.'

'One needs to be on medication for the rest of one's life.'

'Complications are inevitable.'

Like many things I was taught in medical school, these statements have fortunately turned out to be wrong. In recent years, there has been a gradual realisation that type 2 diabetes can be well controlled and, in many cases, put into remission, not with some new expensive medication, but rather an adjustment to the way we eat.

Like many things in life, it is pretty obvious when you think about it. Type 2 diabetes is a disease of carbohydrate intolerance; in other words, the body does not metabolise the sugar and starches we eat, leading to a rise in the blood sugar level. We have known this for decades. Yet in that time, what has been the recommended diet for type 2 diabetes? A low-fat, high-carbohydrate diet!

Such has been our (faulty) obsession with the evils of dietary fats, we have completely lost sight of the real evil – sugar and processed carbohydrates. Our diets have become full of cheap, sweet-tasting, processed and ultra-processed foods.

The result? We have become fatter and sicker.

If you have a disease where you don't tolerate carbohydrates, surely the obvious solution is to avoid carbohydrates. Many thousands of people with type 2 diabetes or pre-diabetes are now doing just that, with remarkable results. In most studies and in our surveys of Defeat Diabetes members, more than half of those with type 2 diabetes put their diabetes into remission. In other words, their HbA1c (the indicator of blood sugar levels) dipped below 6.5 per cent, the threshold for the diagnosis of type 2 diabetes.

Reducing the amount of carbohydrates and increasing healthy fats and proteins in your diet can lead to reduced appetite, increased energy, better sleep, improved exercise tolerance, loss of body fat and reversal of fatty liver. It has also been shown to have a beneficial effect on many chronic diseases, including metabolic syndrome and hypertension.

I became aware of the benefits of eating this way

through my own health experience, as well as the subsequent experiences of many friends and patients. I have since made it my mission to spread the word so others can also experience remission of their type 2 diabetes or reversal of their pre-diabetes.

Recently, I worked with a team of doctors and dietitians to produce an online and app-based program, Defeat Diabetes, which has now been used by thousands of Australians to improve their blood glucose control. *The Diabetes Plan* is based on similar principles and will introduce you to the idea that reducing carbohydrate intake can benefit almost everyone, but particularly those with type 2 diabetes, pre-diabetes or any chronic disease.

This book you are holding in your hands will give you all the information you need to change your eating habits and improve your health. I will explain how processed nutrient-hollow foods have caused a diabesity epidemic and how a diet of real, nutrient-dense food is the key to our wellbeing. We'll look at the carb content of ingredients and reveal which foods should be avoided and what to enjoy instead. We'll also bust some of the common myths around low-carb diets. Plus, there are real-life case studies to educate and inspire.

So, what are you waiting for? Let's go and defeat diabetes.

Learn more

To learn more about my
Defeat Diabetes Program,
scan the QR code.

1

A play in two acts

ACT 1: 'No hope'

Scene: A doctor's surgery

Doctor *(with a grave look on his face)*: Hello Mrs [name deleted], I have the results of your blood tests and I am afraid I have some bad news for you – you have type 2 diabetes.

Patient: That's terrible. My father had type 2 diabetes and I remember what it did to his health. What can I do?

Doctor: Well, I'm afraid that type 2 diabetes is a chronic progressive disease so all we can do is try and reduce the impact of this condition on your health by giving you medications. I want to start you on some tablets straight away.

Patient: But what about diet? I have heard that reducing carbohydrates is a good idea if you have diabetes.

Doctor: No, there is no need to reduce carbohydrates. The important thing is to stick to a low-fat diet. You can have as many carbohydrates as you like – we'll just adjust your medications accordingly.

Intermission

Soft drinks and chocolates served.

ACT 2: 'Hope'

Doctor *(with grave look on his face)*: Hello Mrs [name deleted], I have the results of your blood tests and your blood glucose levels are raised. You have type 2 diabetes.

Patient: That's terrible. My father had type 2 diabetes and I remember what it did to his health. What can I do?

Doctor: Your father was probably just treated with medications and would have developed some of the complications of diabetes. Now we understand that restricting your carbohydrate intake can improve control of your blood glucose, and even put your diabetes into remission.

Patient: I will do anything to avoid the complications that my father developed.

Doctor: Well, before we go down the track of treating with medications, let's get you on a low-carbohydrate diet and see if we can put your diabetes into remission. At the very least, we will improve control of your blood sugars.

Patient: That would be wonderful. I've gone from having no hope to having some hope after all.

The end.

We all need hope in our lives. And people diagnosed with type 2 diabetes can now have that hope. Hope that with a low-carbohydrate diet, they can get their type 2 diabetes under control. Hope that they can avoid the complications that occur as a result of persistent high blood sugars, including blindness, amputations, heart disease, kidney disease and dementia.

Type 2 diabetes no longer needs to be considered a chronic progressive disease.

Let's meet Robert.

Hi Peter,

Three months ago, I was diagnosed with type 2 diabetes with an HbA1c of 16.8. I tried the meds, but they made me very ill. I came across your story on the ABC and decided to follow your diet. In three months, I have reversed my type 2 diabetes (HbA1c = 5.7), and

I've dropped 15kg with no exercise other than working. Giving up sugar and carbs was the best decision I've made for my health in years. My doctor has been promoting my results as he was very sceptical in the beginning.

A few months later . . .

Hi Peter, thought I would send you an update. I'm still travelling along well. My latest HbA1c was 4.8. I've dropped 21kg now, gone from size 42 pants down to size 33, feeling better and still enjoying my food. I get lots of compliments and questions about what I eat, and I've been able to educate a lot of the places where I eat on providing low-carb options.

Pretty impressive, Robert.

My own story is not quite that dramatic, but let me tell you about it because it will help you understand why I am so passionate about this way of eating.

2

My story

'How are you, doc? Are you well?'

If someone had asked me that in 2012, I would have said, 'Yeah, I'm good, thanks. Pretty healthy.' I was living in Liverpool in the UK, working at the famous football club there. I had just turned 60, I had a good diet, or what I thought was a good diet, and I exercised regularly. Yep, pretty healthy!

The reality was that I wasn't quite as healthy as I thought. For a start, I had a family history of type 2 diabetes. In fact, my father had developed it at that very age. I was overweight, borderline obese. Like many men my age, I'd probably put on half a kilogram a year for the last 30 years and was now about 15kg overweight.

I was metabolically unhealthy as well. I had high triglyceride (blood fat) levels, high insulin levels and I'd had a condition known as fatty liver for at least ten years. Whenever I had a blood test, it would come back as 'consistent with fatty liver'. I didn't really understand what fatty liver was and I figured I was on a low-fat diet so I was on the right track. Like a typical doctor, I ignored it.

I wasn't as healthy as I thought and, in retrospect, I was clearly pre-diabetic.

Around that time, my colleague from South Africa, Professor Tim Noakes, was suggesting that we had got nutrition all wrong. It wasn't fat that was the problem in our diet – it was sugar and carbohydrates. He had managed to reverse his type 2 diabetes (which he developed despite being an avid runner with multiple marathons to his name) by changing from a low-fat diet to a low-carbohydrate diet. He said he felt so much better, his running improved and his blood sugar level had stabilised.

Tim is a really smart guy, and I thought, 'I need to look into this,' so I bought a book, *Good Calories, Bad Calories* by Gary Taubes. It blew me away. Not only did Gary speak about the relative merits of fats and carbohydrates, but he also talked about the politics of how the low-fat movement had won out over the low-carb movement back in the 1960s and 70s.

I was really disturbed by this book. I remember sitting down on the edge of my bed and thinking, 'No, this can't be true; we couldn't have got this wrong for the past 40 years! We couldn't have had the whole of western society on the wrong diet for four decades.'

Yet all the evidence he provided seemed to indicate just that.

When I finished that book, I read everything I could get my hands on – research articles, newspaper articles, books. The more I read, the more I became convinced that Taubes and Noakes were right – we *had* been on the wrong diet for 40 years. While we were obsessively removing fat from every item of food, we should have been restricting sugar and carbohydrates.

Eventually I decided it was time for an experiment on myself. I decided I would try a low-carb, healthy-fat diet for three months and see what happened.

On day one, I got my blood tests done and weighed myself. Then I stopped eating all sugars and starches – no bread, rice, pasta, potato, cereal, fruit juice, starchy vegetables. No margarine or vegetable oils. No processed foods at all.

What did I eat instead? I went back to eating the way that my grandparents had probably eaten – meat, fish, eggs, butter, full-fat milk and cream, non-starchy vegetables, olive oil and nuts. The only fruit I had was berries. I drank water, tea and coffee, and an occasional glass of red wine. My indulgence was a square of dark chocolate after dinner every night.

And what happened?

The first thing was that I stopped being hungry. Instead of having my usual cereal in the morning and then feeling hungry only a couple of hours later, I had bacon, eggs and avocado for breakfast and did not feel hungry all day. I went from eating three meals and three snacks a day to eating two meals a day – and I still eat two meals to this very day.

Then I started to lose weight. I initially thought it was just fluid, but it kept coming off.

Other things started to happen. I began to feel more energetic, I felt able to concentrate better, I didn't feel tired during the afternoon, my sleep at night improved, my snoring reduced and my exercise capacity increased. All while eating delicious low-carb, healthy-fat meals with no limit on the amount of food I could enjoy.

For breakfast, I would have eggs, bacon and avocado, and sometimes mushrooms, tomato or sausages, or I would have a cold breakfast of full-fat Greek yoghurt with a mixture of nuts, seeds and some berries. If I needed a snack during the day, I would eat some nuts or a piece of cheese. In the evening, I would have meat or fish with lots of green vegetables such as broccoli, beans, spinach, zucchini, as well as cauliflower and carrots. If I still felt hungry, I would have some berries with full-fat cream. I enjoyed every meal and I never felt hungry.

So, what happened? At the end of the three months, I had lost 13kg despite never feeling hungry and eating as much as I liked. The more fat I ate, the more fat

I lost! I remember feeling quite guilty. I thought losing weight was supposed to be hard, yet I found it easy and so enjoyable.

As well as the weight loss, when I repeated my blood tests, all my metabolic abnormalities had resolved. My triglycerides had gone back to normal, my insulin level had gone back to normal, and that fatty liver that I'd had for ten years had completely disappeared. My liver function tests had returned to normal and have remained so ever since.

In the space of three months, I had:

▶ Reduced my appetite
▶ Lost 13kg in weight
▶ Increased energy
▶ Improved sleep
▶ Decreased triglycerides
▶ Normalised insulin levels
▶ Resolved fatty liver

There was one negative – I needed a new wardrobe, as I had gone down two sizes in clothes. I figured that was a small price to pay.

Everyone who saw me noticed the difference immediately, and always asked what I had done to effect such a change. When something like that happens in your life, I guess you have two choices: you can either say, 'I'm okay, mate' and keep it to yourself or you feel some sort of obligation to tell people what has happened. So that's what I did.

I soon became a vocal advocate for this type of lifestyle, the low-carb lifestyle. I started to give talks and write articles. In 2015, I started the not-for-profit charity SugarByHalf, with the aim of reducing the amount of added sugar eaten per day by one-half. In 2019, I was approached to write a book and wrote *A Fat Lot of Good*, which was on the bestseller list for a number of weeks. Then finally, in January 2021, we launched Defeat Diabetes (for more on the program, see Chapter 16).

I consider myself extremely lucky.

If I had not heard about low-carb from Tim Noakes, I would have continued the way I was going. I have no doubt that, given I was clearly pre-diabetic at the time, I would have developed type 2 diabetes by now, and probably have developed some of the complications associated with that condition.

I reckon I dodged a bullet!

3

Understanding
diabetes

What is diabetes?

Diabetes is a condition associated with raised levels of glucose, a type of sugar, in your blood. There are a number of different types of diabetes, but we are primarily interested in the most common – type 2 diabetes.

What are the different types of diabetes?

▶ Type 1 diabetes is an autoimmune condition that tends to affect younger people. The body attacks the insulin-producing beta cells of the pancreas, destroying them. Treatment requires regular insulin injections because of the body's inability to produce insulin.

- ▶ Type 2 diabetes accounts for 90 per cent of those with diabetes and usually occurs later in life. It is often associated with obesity and is caused by insulin resistance. It is treated with medication and lifestyle measures, such as a low-carb diet.
- ▶ Gestational diabetes develops during pregnancy and affects 12–14 per cent of pregnant women. Approximately half the women who have gestational diabetes go on to develop type 2 diabetes.
- ▶ Pre-diabetes is a group of conditions such as metabolic syndrome, non-alcoholic fatty liver disease (NAFLD) and obesity, all of which are linked to insulin resistance. They are thought to lead in many instances to the development of type 2 diabetes.
- ▶ LADA (or Latent Auto-immune Diabetes in Adults) is, like type 1 diabetes, an auto-immune condition, where the body attacks insulin-secreting cells within the pancreas. Those with LADA eventually require insulin injections.

To understand type 2 diabetes, let's have a look at what happens when we eat a meal containing carbohydrates.

When we eat food containing sugars or starches, such as bread, rice, pasta or cereal, the body breaks down that carbohydrate to the simple sugar – glucose. Glucose is then absorbed from the gut into the bloodstream.

When glucose is absorbed into the bloodstream, it triggers the release of a hormone called insulin from the pancreas. Insulin acts to drive the glucose out of the bloodstream and into the body's tissues, initially to the liver and ultimately throughout the body.

When there is not enough insulin produced or, more commonly, the body has become resistant to the effect of insulin (known as insulin resistance), the blood glucose levels stay elevated. When this level rises above a certain threshold, the diagnosis of type 2 diabetes is made.

Diagnosis of type 2 diabetes

Symptoms such as excessive thirst, excessive urination, blurred vision, fatigue, weight loss or recurrent infections such as thrush may be suggestive of the diagnosis of type 2 diabetes. However, in the early stages of the disease, there are frequently no specific symptoms. The diagnosis of type 2 diabetes is usually made on the basis of a blood test, either the fasting blood glucose or the HbA1c, which is a measure of the average blood glucose levels over the previous three months. A slightly raised blood level is diagnosed as pre-diabetes. If the fasting blood glucose is greater than 7.0, or the HbA1c is 6.5 or above, then the diagnosis of type 2 diabetes is made:

	Fasting blood glucose (FBG)	HbA1c	HbA1c
	(mmol/L)	(%)	(mmol/mol)
Normal	<5.6	<6.0	<42
Pre-diabetes	5.6–6.9	6.0–6.4	42–47
Type 2 diabetes	7.0 or above	6.5 or above	48 or above

How does insulin resistance cause diabetes?

Insulin resistance is a key factor in the development of type 2 diabetes and other chronic diseases. If you eat a diet high in sugar or high-carbohydrate foods, your body gradually requires more and more insulin to control your blood sugar level. This is known as insulin resistance.

As insulin is also a fat-storage hormone (it converts excess glucose to fat), these high levels of insulin lead to increased fat storage and salt retention, among other health issues.

Eventually, the pancreas simply cannot produce the insulin needed to counteract the sugar. Blood glucose levels start to rise, and the result is type 2 diabetes.

What is metabolic syndrome?

Metabolic syndrome is often regarded as a step along the way to the diagnosis of type 2 diabetes. Metabolic syndrome is a combination of:

- ▶ High blood pressure
- ▶ High blood glucose
- ▶ Obesity
- ▶ High triglycerides
- ▶ Low HDL cholesterol

It is associated with insulin resistance and is regarded as a major risk factor for type 2 diabetes and cardiovascular disease.

Why is type 2 diabetes such a problem?

While type 2 diabetes may not be the most common direct cause of death, it is arguably the most important indirect cause. Excess levels of glucose in the blood cause progressive damage to blood vessels, both the large blood vessels (macrovascular), leading to heart disease and strokes, and small blood vessels, leading to blindness, dementia (including Alzheimer's), kidney and nerve damage. It is, in many cases, directly related to the three most common causes of death – cardiovascular (heart, vessel disease), dementia (including Alzheimer's) and cerebrovascular disease (strokes).

People with diabetes have a significantly higher risk of:

▶ Cardiovascular disease – angina, heart attacks, strokes
▶ Dementia and Alzheimer's disease – which has been described as 'type 3 diabetes'
▶ Amputations due to lower limb damage, such as ulcers
▶ Blindness (diabetes is the leading cause of blindness in adults)
▶ Kidney disease and kidney failure (dialysis)
▶ Skin infections, both bacterial and fungal
▶ Nerve damage, such as numbness and loss of feeling

Monitoring type 2 diabetes

Once you are diagnosed with type 2 diabetes, it is important to monitor your blood glucose levels. Your doctor will test your fasting blood glucose level every three to six months and will also test your HbA1c, which as mentioned is a guide to your previous three months' blood glucose levels.

In addition to your regular blood tests, it is possible to easily measure your blood glucose at any time. This has traditionally been done using a drop of blood obtained with a lancet pinprick of one's finger and then measuring the level with the use of small blood glucose strips and a blood glucose meter.

More recently, the use of continuous glucose monitors (CGM) has revolutionised the management of type 1 diabetes, and they will ultimately be available to those with type 2 diabetes. The CGM gives immediate feedback on the effect of any food you eat. It is a great educational tool to enable you to determine which specific foods lead to excessive glucose levels.

These CGMs are attached painlessly to the skin and give a continuous glucose reading. They currently need to be replaced every two weeks, but that period will hopefully lengthen in the near future.

Using a continuous glucose monitor (CGM)

CGMs have transformed the management of diabetes. They remove the guesswork about the impact of specific foods on your blood glucose levels, allowing you to personally tailor your diet to your metabolism.

A CGM is a small sensor that you attach to your stomach or the back of your upper arm, which then communicates wirelessly with your phone. You will be provided with a real-time readout of your blood sugar levels without the need to prick your finger. This will allow you to identify any foods that cause spiking in your blood sugar. By avoiding those foods in future, you will be able to achieve excellent control of your diabetes, significantly reducing your risk of future complications.

Your main goal should be to achieve a 'flat' graph. If you see a spike in your blood sugar occurring soon after a meal, you should identify what caused this and understand that, at least for you, that food is not a healthy choice.

Low-carb meals should cause little, if any, increase in your blood sugar levels. You may find, for example, that a breakfast of eggs and bacon doesn't impact your sugar level at all, while eggs on white toast does.

Example of a 'flat' blood sugar level associated with low-carb eating.

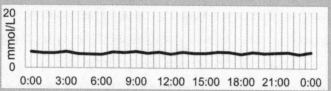

Example of a spike in blood glucose associated with high-carb food. This food should not be consumed again.

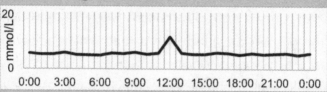

The most readily available CGM in Australia is the Freestyle Libre. Most people only need to purchase one sensor, as two weeks is sufficient to determine which foods need to be avoided. If your mobile phone is not compatible, you can purchase a 'Reader' separately.

FAQs

Can I exercise with the sensor on?
Yes. The sensor is painless, and you won't even know it is there. You can shower as normal, and even swim, so long as it is for less than 30 minutes.

Is it painful?

No. While there is a small needle that breaks the skin, it is completely painless. The continuous glucose monitor also removes the need to prick your finger, which can be uncomfortable.

What ranges should I set for my blood glucose levels?

It is reasonable to enter a target reference range between 3.9 and 7.0 mmol/L, however, a steady blood glucose graph is most important. If you have a history of poorly controlled diabetes, you should seek further advice from your GP.

Why can't I get a 'flat' blood glucose reading?

Besides hidden carbs in food, there are several reasons why your blood sugar levels may not be stable, which can include an illness or infection. If your blood sugar control suddenly worsens, it is recommended you see your doctor. Other factors that can cause blood sugar levels to rise include hot showers, exercise and corticosteroid medications (such as prednisone), which are often used for inflammatory conditions.

What should I do if I get a low reading?

If you have a finger-prick blood glucose meter

available, use this to confirm the accuracy of any low readings.

While low blood sugar levels can be dangerous, many patients with low readings do not have any problems. In fact, if you have been on a very low-carbohydrate diet for at least several weeks and are not feeling unwell, you may not need to do anything at all about a low reading. On the other hand, if you have symptoms such as unusual hunger, headache, dizziness, fast heart rate or nausea, you should consume about 15 grams of fast-acting carbohydrates (equivalent to about six or seven jellybeans) and speak to your doctor.

Note that problems with low blood sugar levels are very unlikely unless you are taking certain diabetic medications, such as sulphonylureas or insulin. Metformin, the most common diabetic medication, does not cause low blood sugar levels, by itself.

Learn more

Scan the QR code to take a short quiz on the Defeat Diabetes website. This quiz will help you discover if you're at risk of developing type 2 diabetes.

4

The diabesity epidemic

The 'Diabesity' epidemic (obesity and type 2 diabetes) is likely to be the biggest epidemic in human history.

Professor Paul Zimmet AO, 2007

We have heard a lot about pandemics and epidemics recently, but the words above from eminent Australian diabetes expert Professor Paul Zimmet ring true.

Let's look at the numbers.

Diabetes

In 2021 the International Diabetes Federation (IDF) released the 10th edition of their *IDF Global Atlas* with updated figures on the incidence and cost of diabetes. It makes for grim reading.

Since the first edition in 2000, the estimated world-wide prevalence of diabetes in adults aged 20–79 years has more than tripled, from an estimated 151 million (4.6 per cent of the global population at the time) to 537 million (10.5 per cent) today. Without sufficient action to address the situation, they are predicting 643 million people will have diabetes by 2030 (11.3 per cent of the population), and if trends continue, the number will jump to a staggering 783 million (12.2 per cent) by 2045.

Globally, more than one in ten adults are now living with diabetes. Moreover, there is a growing list of countries where one in five or even more of the adult population has diabetes. Almost one in two adults with diabetes is unaware they have the condition. An estimated 240 million people are living with undiagnosed diabetes.

Approximately 6.7 million adults aged between 20–79 are estimated to have died as a result of diabetes or its complications in 2021. This corresponds to 12.2 per cent of global deaths from all causes in this age group. Approximately one-third (32.6 per cent) of all deaths from diabetes occur in people of working age (under the age of 60). This corresponds to 11.8 per cent of total global deaths in people under 60.

The overall direct cost of diabetes worldwide is A\$1.344 trillion (or A\$1,344 billion), a 316 per cent increase in cost over the last 15 years.

The Australian picture is no better.

One-and-a-half million Australians aged between 20–79 have diabetes, which equates to a prevalence of 8.2 per cent of the population, and 280 Australians are diagnosed with diabetes every day; that's over 100,000 annually. Another approximately 400,000 are thought to be undiagnosed. The annual number of diabetes-related deaths is over 20,000. The annual cost of diabetes in Australia, including direct health costs and government subsidies, is estimated to be A$19 billion.

Obesity

Obesity is associated with a higher mortality rate and increases the likelihood of many chronic diseases including type 2 diabetes, and Australia has one of the highest rates of obesity in the world. Two-thirds of all adult Australians are overweight (36 per cent) or obese (31 per cent). The obesity rate has increased from 19 per cent in 1995. It is slightly more prevalent in males than females and is more common in older age groups.

A quarter of all Australian children and adolescents aged five to 17 are overweight, with 8.1 per cent obese, almost double the figure from a generation ago.

Where have we gone wrong?

A generation or two ago, seeing an obese person in the street or at the beach was a rarity. Likewise, it was unusual to see a patient in clinic with type 2 diabetes. In fact, the condition was originally known as adult-onset or mature-onset diabetes, until they had to change the name because so many younger people were developing it. The rate of incidence of both diabetes and obesity has increased dramatically in the past 40 years.

Why?

Some people blame lack of exercise; however, the amount of exercise we do now is not dissimilar to a generation or two ago, except that then it was more occupation-related and now it is more leisure-related. Certainly not enough difference to explain the increase in obesity and diabetes.

What *has* changed dramatically is what we eat and drink. Our grandparents' generation ate a diet consisting of meat, poultry, eggs, dairy, fruit and vegetables. They cooked with butter, beef tallow, duck fat or lard and they drank water, beer and copious amounts of tea.

Then we were told – wrongly, as it has turned out – that cholesterol and saturated fat were the cause of the increasing rates of heart disease. We were advised by government-appointed committees producing dietary guidelines that we needed to reduce the cholesterol and saturated fat (all that butter, fat and lard) in our diet and replace them with carbohydrates and polyunsaturated fats (vegetable oils).

The food industry saw this as an opportunity, and produced a vast array of 'low-fat' foods. However, when they removed the fat from foods, they discovered that much of the flavour also disappeared, so they came up with a brilliant (for their profits) solution – replace the fat with sugar. So the recommended low-fat foods were actually low-fat/high-sugar foods.

The result has been a disaster: we have just got fatter and sicker.

Processed, take-away or junk foods and ready-to-eat meals now fill our shopping baskets. Over 80 per cent of processed foods contain added sugar, often disguised by using one of the 50-odd names the industry uses for sugar.

Foods such as 'low-fat' fruit yoghurts, cereals, muesli bars, sauces, mayonnaise, bread and most packaged ready-to-heat meals are full of added sugar. Take-away foods are cooked with re-used vegetable oil and are full of sugar. The food industry has succeeded in getting us all addicted to sweetness – sweet is the new normal.

Calories out, nutrient-density in

Calories in, calories out. Calories, calories, calories. That's all some people ever focus on. But we don't eat calories; we eat food.

Many foods are nutrient-hollow – lacking any nutrients such as vitamins and minerals. It is important to focus on eating nutrient-dense foods rather than foods with little to no nutritional value.

Common nutrient-hollow and nutrient-dense foods

Nutrient-hollow foods	Nutrient-dense foods
Sugar	Eggs
Foods with added sugars, including many foods labelled 'low-fat'	Full-fat dairy, including butter, milk, cheese
White flour	Meat – beef, lamb, pork, chicken
Cakes	Oily fish – salmon, sardines, mackerel
Biscuits, cookies, crisps	Shellfish – oysters, prawns, mussels
Confectionery	Liver and other organ meats
Ice cream	Nuts – particularly almonds, macadamias
Margarine	Olive oil, lard, ghee
Vegetable (seed) oils	Mushrooms
Soft drinks	Seaweed
Fruit-flavoured drinks	Avocado
Beer	Green vegetables, especially broccoli, spinach
	Cacao – 70+ per cent dark chocolate

> Nutrient-hollow food is fine in small amounts, but most of what you eat should be nutrient-dense.

'The diabetes diet'

Given that type 2 diabetes is a disease where one does not tolerate carbohydrates, what do you think the recommended diet (based on fraudulent research and a corrupt industry) for those with type 2 diabetes has been for the past 50 years?

A high-carbohydrate, low-fat diet.

Let me say that again – a *high-carbohydrate, low-fat diet.*

Such has been our obsession with reducing fat intake that we have got diabetes management totally the wrong way around. A high-carbohydrate diet is the *worst* thing you can do for your diabetes. It perpetuates high blood glucose levels, which is exactly what we want to avoid in order to minimise any long-term damage to our eyes, heart, kidneys, nerves and legs.

Fortunately, people are starting to realise the error of our ways – some would say the biggest mistake in medical history – and are using a low-carbohydrate diet in type 2 diabetes management with remarkable results.

Inflammation

We now understand that chronic low-grade inflammation is a major cause of most of the chronic diseases that are so prevalent in the modern world. These include atherosclerosis, type 2 diabetes, heart disease, stroke, asthma and other respiratory diseases. Even mental illnesses such as anxiety and depression are now thought to be closely associated with inflammation.

In diseases associated with acute inflammation, the standard treatment involves the use of anti-inflammatory medications, but the most successful management has involved modifying lifestyle factors, particularly diet.

Dietary factors that promote inflammation include sugar, processed carbohydrates, vegetable (seed) oils, alcohol and processed meats. It seems that some but not all individuals find specific foods, such as gluten or dairy, inflammatory as well.

The management of these chronic diseases associated with chronic low-grade inflammation is now focusing on removing sugars, processed carbohydrates and vegetable oils from the diets of those suffering, with encouraging results. In diseases such as Parkinson's disease, Alzheimer's disease, inflammatory bowel disease and mental illness, to name just a few, research has shown dietary measures to be at least, if not more, effective than the traditional use of medications, with many additional positive effects to overall health, and reduced adverse effects when compared to drugs.

Learn more

You can learn more about how chronic inflammation affects type 2 diabetes and many other chronic diseases through my Defeat Diabetes online webinar. Scan the QR code to watch.

5

Defeat diabetes

Now that we understand how prevalent and potentially serious type 2 diabetes is, let's look at how we can manage it. There are two main objectives in the management of diabetes. The first is to maintain a low average blood glucose level, as demonstrated by a reduced HbA1c level, and the second is to avoid short-term spikes and fluctuations in blood glucose levels.

Contrary to long-held opinion that there is no way of putting type 2 diabetes into remission, recent evidence shows that there are potentially three different methods that can be effective. However, only one of those is practical and realistic.

The first method is bariatric surgery, which is the name given to a group of surgical procedures that reduce the capacity of the gastrointestinal tract to absorb nutrients from food. This may involve reducing the size of, or bypassing, the stomach. It is a fairly radical procedure usually only undertaken on morbidly obese patients when other methods have failed, and significant medical problems are associated with their obesity. It has been shown to be effective in controlling blood glucose levels but is associated with frequent side effects, such as 'dumping syndrome', which leads to nausea and dizziness, low blood glucose and vomiting.

The second effective measure for both weight loss and diabetes control is a low-calorie diet. Diets of around 800 calories, often in the form of liquid shakes, have been shown by Professor Roy Taylor at Newcastle University in the UK to be effective in the management of type 2 diabetes and weight loss. Other studies also support the use of a very low-calorie approach in managing type 2 diabetes.

The problem with low-calorie diets and the reason why they almost always fail is hunger. More specifically, you become 'hangry' – hungry and angry. It is almost impossible to sustain a very low-calorie diet, such as 800 calories, for more than a few weeks due to constant hunger. It is not sustainable (or enjoyable) to drink shakes alone on a long-term basis.

The other problem with a low-calorie diet is that your body responds by going into 'starvation mode' and slowing down its base rate of metabolism. Then when you eventually break the diet and resume normal calorie intake, you still have a slow metabolism and put on all the weight you have lost, plus some!

The third way to both lose weight and improve your diabetes control is with a low-carbohydrate diet. For a condition like type 2 diabetes, in which your body does not tolerate carbohydrates, reducing your carbohydrates makes a lot of sense. You avoid the sudden spikes after eating a carbohydrate meal, and you maintain an average lower blood glucose level. The biggest advantage is that you are not hungry.

Carbohydrates make you hungry; protein and fats make you feel full (satiated). Because of that feeling of satiety, there is not the constant desire to snack and you need to eat less often, as little as once or twice a day.

Learn more

In 2022, I discussed how a low-carb diet could achieve remission with Dr David Unwin, a UK GP who has been studying the impact of carbohydrate restriction on his patients with type 2 diabetes. To watch our conversation, scan the QR code.

Show me the evidence!

There have now been numerous randomised control trials (RCTs), the highest level of scientific evidence, which have shown low-carb diets to be superior to low-fat diets in the management of type 2 diabetes.

A meta-analysis – where the results of multiple scientific studies are combined and analysed – on the effect of low-carbohydrate diets (LCDs) on rates of remission of diabetes, was published in *The BMJ* – arguably the world's most prestigious medical journal – in January 2021.

This systematic review included 23 trials, including unpublished HbA1c and medication use data from five trials and concluded:

> compared with (mostly low-fat) control diets, on the basis of moderate certainty evidence at six months, LCDs were associated with a large (32 per cent) increase in remission of diabetes. Large and clinically important improvements in weight loss, triglycerides and insulin resistance were also seen, without adverse events.

Another systematic review of RCTs, published in the *Journal of Nutritional Science* in 2021, looked at whether restricting calorie intake as well as reducing carbohydrates is an advantage over a low-carbohydrate diet with unlimited calories.

This paper found 15 RCTs that met the inclusion criteria. Nine of the 15 studies utilised LCDs with moderate or unrestricted energy intake, while the other six utilised low-energy diets (LED) of less than 1200 calories per day, with all except one incorporating meal replacements as part of a commercial weight loss program. Both types of diets produced significant weight loss and reduction of HbA1c in their trials.

The interesting result was that trials that restricted energy intake at 12 and 24 months were not superior to those that allowed unlimited low-carbohydrate feeding. The two studies reporting the largest changes by 12 and 24 months involved low-carbohydrate diets with unrestricted or moderate energy restriction. The most effective intervention at 12 and 24 months involved a very low-carbohydrate (ketogenic) diet with unlimited calorie intake.

The main message from this study is that restricting energy intake in the context of a low-carbohydrate diet is of no added advantage.

This has enormous consequences, as it means that reducing carbohydrate intake does not have to be associated with calorie restriction. It is extremely difficult to adhere to a low-calorie diet, such as the 800 calories per day in many of these studies, due to the constant hunger experienced by the participants. The second issue is that all but one of the low-calorie diets consisted of meal replacements, which are not sustainable in the long-term.

So this review shows that restricting carbohydrate intake is sufficient, without having to restrict calorie intake and without needing to use meal replacements.

What about online or app-based programs? Can they be effective?

Online programs similar to Defeat Diabetes have been established for several years in both the UK and the USA. The UK program has seen more than 400,000 people undertake a low-carb program, with a study by Saslow et al. in 2018 finding those who completed ten weeks of this program reduced their HbA1c from an average of 9.2 per cent to 7.1 per cent. Over a quarter of the participants reduced their HbA1c to below the diabetes threshold, and 40 per cent reduced their diabetes medications. These participants also lost an average of 6.9 per cent of their body weight.

In the USA, a remote care model run by Virta Health has also proven to be successful. While reducing and eliminating glycemic control medications, Virta patients lowered HbA1c by 1.3 per cent on average after one year and improved insulin resistance. Sixty per cent of patients enrolled for one year attained an HbA1c below 6.5 per cent without the use of diabetes medications other than metformin. Their patients also lost weight (12 per cent of body weight) and improved hypertension, measures of inflammation and cardio-vascular risk factors.

And then . . .

So what if I succeed and manage to improve control of my blood glucose levels and even put my type 2 diabetes into remission? Will I notice anything different?

You almost certainly will notice a number of changes – apart from the reading on your blood glucose meter! We can divide the possible effects into short-term and longer-term.

Short-term

In the short-term, excessive fatigue and lethargy should gradually lift, and you will have more energy. Your sleep may improve in both quality and quantity. If you have been suffering from sleep apnoea, this is likely to improve.

You won't feel as tired when you wake up as you did previously. You will probably feel more mentally alert and start thinking more clearly. Any brain fog will noticeably lift.

You are likely to begin losing weight almost immediately. Many who turn to a low-carb diet lose between 0.5 and 1kg each week for the first few weeks.

Type 2 diabetes is frequently associated with low mood, including depression and anxiety. This will often start to improve soon after getting your blood glucose levels under control. Dietary changes have been shown to be equally as effective as medication in the treatment of depression.

Many chronic medical conditions are associated with chronic low-grade inflammation throughout the body, and a diet low in carbohydrates and vegetable oils can reduce the amount of inflammation, with improvement in conditions such as arthritis, gout, autoimmune diseases, PCOS and many others.

I'm always surprised by how many people approach me after changing to a low-carb diet to say how their gut symptoms, which they have often not even mentioned to their doctor, have improved. Symptoms such as bloating, abdominal discomfort and intermittent diarrhoea are frequently eliminated by a changing of diet.

Type 2 diabetes is associated with an increase in infections, often skin or urinary, probably due to impaired immunity. Improved blood glucose control is likely to reduce the incidence of infection.

In the past couple of years, it has become evident that those with type 2 diabetes have been both more likely to test positive for Covid-19 and be more likely to experience serious consequences.

Longer-term

The major reason for wanting to improve blood glucose control is to prevent the development of the serious long-term consequences of type 2 diabetes – cardio-vascular, eye, kidney, neurological and vascular complications.

Improved blood glucose control reduces risk factors for cardiovascular diseases such as heart attacks, angina, heart failure and strokes. Cardiovascular disease is the number-one killer in Australia and poor blood glucose control is a major risk factor. Some heart specialists go so far as to say that everyone who has a heart attack has underlying impaired glucose control, many previously undiagnosed.

Diabetes is the most common cause of blindness, due to disease of the retina. Good blood glucose control will nearly always prevent the development of blindness.

Diabetes is the most common cause of kidney failure resulting in the need for dialysis or kidney transplant. The small blood vessels of the kidneys become damaged and affect the efficiency of the filter function. This can usually be prevented with good blood glucose control.

Nerve cells can be damaged by excessive exposure to glucose, resulting in tingling, loss of sensation or pain, often initially in the feet. Many different areas of the body can be affected by diabetic nerve damage. Nerve damage caused by high blood glucose levels can cause men to have difficulty in getting an erection. Frequently, improved blood glucose control will result in improved nerve function.

Vascular disease secondary to poor blood glucose control can affect the arteries of the leg, resulting in impaired blood supply at the ends of the limb. This can lead initially to the development of an ulcer, which subsequently may fail to heal and ultimately require amputation of the foot. Diabetes is the most common cause of amputation of the lower limb. Sadly, some patients require multiple amputations as the disease spreads up their leg. Yet lower leg circulation can improve with better blood glucose control.

As mentioned above, there is a strong relationship between diabetes and mental health, and improving blood glucose control can lead to a significant improvement in conditions such as depression and anxiety.

Intermittent fasting

Reducing carbohydrate intake minimises the production of the fat-storage hormone insulin. Another way of reducing this insulin secretion is by fasting.

Dr Jason Fung, co-author of *The Complete Guide to Fasting*, lists seven advantages of fasting:

1. Simplicity
2. Affordability
3. Convenience
4. Cheat days
5. Powerful effects
6. Flexibility
7. Versatility – it can be added to any diet

There are certain groups who should not try fasting, including pregnant and breastfeeding women, children and the elderly. For everyone else, there do not appear to be any negative health outcomes and there seem to be plenty of positives.

The different types of fasting include:

▶ 12/24/36 hours fasting
▶ The 5:2 diet
▶ Time-restricted eating (TRE)

Each of these seem to be effective. Even though we don't consider it to be 'fasting', we all fast overnight and break our fast with 'breakfast'. That might involve ten to 12 hours without eating. A popular fasting regimen is to extend that fast to 14–16 hours by eating an early dinner and late breakfast.

The popular TRE fits all one's food intake into a six- to eight-hour period, with the resultant 16- to 18-hour fast. For example, for those eating two meals a day, one could have the first meal at midday and the second at 6 pm, which gives you a six-hour eating window and a daily 18-hour fast.

Some advocate alternate-day fasting or fasting on one or two days per week. The very popular 5:2 diet involves eating small amounts of food on two days a week and normal intake the other five days.

The initial reaction of most people when some type of fasting is suggested is: 'I couldn't do that, I would get too hungry.' Surprisingly, however, most people manage to fast very easily and are surprised at how long they can go without eating solids. Once you're off the high-carb blood sugar rollercoaster and eating unprocessed food high in good fats, your hunger stabilises so TRE is absolutely possible.

There is increasing evidence of the benefits of fasting for weight loss, improved insulin sensitivity and even type 2 diabetes.

It's important to maintain hydration while fasting, so drink plenty of water, black coffee, green tea or bone broth, all of which are allowed in a fast.

CASE STUDY | Rachael Hamilton

Weight loss: 5.9kg in three months
Fasting blood glucose: Down from 6.4 to 5.4
Age: 55

Summary: For Rachael from Brisbane, weight had never been an issue, but after her husband, Phil, was diagnosed with terminal brain cancer, her world was thrown into disarray. Sitting by Phil's bedside for almost two years, her own health took second place. When Phil passed away, the grief was all-consuming, but she knew she had to be there for her children.

After a thorough health check, Rachael was shocked to learn she had pre-diabetes, but a friend recommended the Defeat Diabetes Program and she's not looked back. After just three months on the program, Rachael has reached her goal weight, and she's no longer in the range for pre-diabetes.

Story: I've been relatively fit all my life. I used to be a long-distance runner, I've always trained and been very healthy, and weight had never been an issue.

In August 2019, my husband, Phil, was diagnosed with terminal brain cancer. I went from training at least two days a week and 'clean' eating to being at the hospital every day, sitting by his bedside.

As his full-time carer, my lifestyle became sedentary for the next two years, and my healthy eating habits went out the window. My diet mainly consisted of hospital food to get me through the long days: hot chocolate, cake, and cheese and ham toasties.

When Phil passed away in May 2021, I went to my GP to have a complete check-up and get my health back on track. When my results came back with pre-diabetes, my GP, who had known me for 25 years, was almost as shocked as I was. I had always been a very fit and healthy person.

The diagnosis was significant, and as Phil was no longer with us, I needed to be sure I'd be around for my children. In hindsight, the signs of pre-diabetes were there, but I put it all down to fatigue and everything else that was going on.

I needed to get back into my groove again, and I needed guidance. When a work friend saw the Defeat Diabetes Program and suggested I give it a go, I thought, what have I got to lose?

The first two weeks were the hardest. I was craving carbs, and I felt tired and sluggish, but after increasing my salt intake (see page 103), my energy levels improved and the cravings started to subside.

The one thing I was stunned to learn was that it was more than just cutting out sugar. Learning how carbohydrates (not just sugars) are the main driver of insulin resistance has been the key to my losing weight and getting my blood sugars lower.

After just three months on the program, I've reached my goal weight, my inflammation has settled down, and my skin, hair and mood are much better. Even my fitness levels are starting to return! Best of all, I'm no longer in the range for pre-diabetes.

I love the food and the way it makes me feel. There's so much variety and change in the menu each week, and I never feel bloated after meals.

I want other people to know about the program, as there may be so many others out there with pre-diabetes who don't even know they have it, especially people my age. It's not just a diet; this is a complete lifestyle change. I can't imagine not eating this way now and am always trying to teach my friends how to eat better. After all, I'm living proof that it works.

6

Restrict carbohydrates

You've already heard a bit about carbohydrates, or carbs as we call them, but you are about to hear a lot more.

Why?

Because restricting carbohydrate intake is the key to maintaining good glucose control if you have type 2 diabetes or pre-diabetes, or if you want to prevent heading in that direction.

What are carbohydrates?

There are two types of carbohydrates – sugars and starches.

Sugars

Sugars are monosaccharides with one simple sugar – glucose, fructose, galactose – or disaccharides with two sugars, such as sucrose (table sugar, a combination of glucose and fructose) and lactose (glucose and galactose), found in dairy foods.

Foods high in sugar include:

- ▶ Sugary beverages, which includes soft drinks, fruit drinks, fruit juices, energy drinks, cordials, flavoured milks and coffees, iced tea, sweet alcoholic drinks
- ▶ Sweet foods including desserts, cakes, biscuits and lollies
- ▶ Processed foods with added sugar, molasses, honey, and other sugars 'in disguise'
- ▶ Fruits that are naturally high in sugar, such as figs and ripe bananas, and dried fruit

Starches

A starch contains a series of multiple glucose molecules joined together by chemical bonds. During the digestion process, they are broken down to glucose and absorbed into the bloodstream. The body does not differentiate between the glucose from a soft drink and the glucose from a piece of white bread; they are all absorbed as the same molecule. The only difference is that the glucose from starch takes a little longer to break down, so you don't get as sharp a spike in blood glucose, but the total amount is the same.

Foods high in starch include:

- ▶ Starchy vegetables – potatoes, sweet potatoes, corn, parsnip, taro
- ▶ Flour – any food made with flour, including bread, crackers, doughnuts, cakes, biscuits, pastries, pasta etc. This is true of wholegrain flours as well, but not true of flours made from nuts or seeds such as almond flour.
- ▶ Wholegrains – rice, barley, oats, quinoa
- ▶ Legumes – beans, peas and lentils

How much carbohydrates should we eat?

There is no set amount of carbs that one should eat – it varies for each of us as individuals, depending on our metabolic health. However, no one should be eating the 200–300 grams of carbs that the average Australian consumes every day. That is a recipe for disaster.

	Carbs – grams/day	Carbs – % calories
Standard Australian diet	200–300	40–60
Moderate-carb	100–130	20–30
Low-carb	30–100	6–20
Very low-carb ('keto')	Less than 30	Less than 6

There is no agreed definition of 'low-carb', but some would say anything under 130g a day is low-carb.

We prefer to think of under 130g as 'moderate-carb', and under 100g as 'low-carb'.

Keto

The term 'keto' or ketogenic diet has become very popular in recent years, and is the number-one diet term searched on Google.

The human body uses two different fuels. It will always use carbohydrates to fuel its various activities if carbs are available. However, if carbs are not available, the body breaks down fat into ketone bodies and uses that as its fuel, hence the term 'keto'.

The body can function perfectly well without carbs, using ketones as its fuel. It is a myth that the body needs 120 grams of carbs a day. What little carbs the body requires can easily be obtained from the small amount of carbohydrates in foods such as vegetables, or the body can make its own glucose from protein or fat, a process known as gluconeogenesis.

How much sugar do we consume?

The World Health Organization recommends no more than six teaspoons per day.

The average Australian consumes about 16 teaspoons of added sugar per day. That number does not account for the 'natural' sugar in fruit and dairy either. Many, especially younger people, consume considerably more. Given that there are 16 teaspoons of added sugar in a 600ml bottle of Coke, it is not surprising that many consume well over 20 teaspoons of extra sugar every day.

We have a long way to go.

Where are we getting our added sugar from?

The biggest contributor to added sugar intake, according to the Australian Bureau of Statistics, is soft drinks and flavoured water, followed by the category of sugar, honey and syrups, then cakes and desserts.

Consumption of added sugars among all Australians

	Percentage of added sugar intake (%)
Soft drinks and flavoured water (not including cordials)	19.4
Sugar, honey and syrups	10.6
Cakes, muffins, scones, cake-type desserts	9.9
Fruit and vegetable juices	6.2
Chocolate and chocolate-based confectionery	5.6

	Percentage of added sugar intake (%)
Cordials	5.4
Sweet biscuits	4.6
Frozen milk products (ice cream, etc.)	4.5
Breakfast cereals, muesli and cereal bars	3.7
Other confectionery	3.0
Sauces, dips and condiments	2.7
Alcoholic beverages	2.6
Flavoured milks and milkshakes	2.5
Jam and lemon spreads, chocolate spreads, sauces	2.4
Yoghurt	2.1

Source: Australian Bureau of Statistics, Australian Health Survey: Consumption of added sugars 2011–12, 2016.

Just over half (52 per cent) of added sugars consumed were from beverages such as those listed below.

Sugar content of popular soft drinks

	Serving size (ml)	Sugar (grams per 100ml)	Sugar (teaspoons per 100ml)
Solo	600	12.1	🥄🥄🥄
Fanta	375	11.2	🥄🥄🥄

	Serving size (ml)	Sugar (grams per 100ml)	Sugar (teaspoons per 100ml)
Red Bull	250	11	🥄🥄🥄
Coca-Cola	375	10.6	🥄🥄🥄
Sprite	600	10.6	🥄🥄🥄
V Energy Drink	500	10.6	🥄🥄🥄
Mother	500	10.4	🥄🥄🥄
Gatorade Fierce Grape	600	6	🥄🥄
Powerade Mountain Blast	600	5.7	🥄🥄
Vitamin Water Essential	500	5.5	🥄🥄
Lipton Ice Tea Peach	500	5.3	🥄🥄

Fruit juices and flavoured milks have always been promoted as healthy, but it turns out they are full of added sugar as well.

Sugar content of fruit juices and flavoured milk

	Serving size (ml)	Sugar (grams per 100ml)	Sugar (teaspoons per 100ml)
Apple juice	240	11	🥄🥄🥄
Fruit drinks	200	9	🥄🥄🥄
Flavoured milk	300	9	🥄🥄🥄
Orange juice	250	8	🥄🥄

An example of commonly used processed foods that are high in sugar are store-bought sauces.

Sugar content of store-bought sauces

	Serving size (ml)	Sugar (grams per serve)	Sugar (teaspoons per serve)
Barbecue	25	12	🥄🥄🥄
Sweet and sour	20	8.5	🥄🥄
Tomato	20	5	🥄
Worcestershire	20	4	🥄

	Serving size (ml)	Sugar (grams per serve)	Sugar (teaspoons per serve)
Satay	20	3.3	
Chilli	20	3	

Fructose

This far we have mainly talked about the problem of glucose and the elevation of blood glucose levels. However, there is another simple sugar that can impact one's health – fructose. Fructose forms one-half (with glucose) of simple table sugar, or sucrose. The main source of fructose is sugar-sweetened drinks (soft drinks, fruit juices, flavoured milks etc.) and confectionery, but it is also the sugar contained in fruit.

Fructose behaves differently from glucose, and is taken up immediately by the liver. Excess fructose is stored as fat in the liver and other organs, including the pancreas. This may lead to a condition known as fatty liver, which is a precursor to type 2 diabetes. As Professor Roy Taylor says, 'Before diabetes, there is a long silent scream from the liver.'

Fruit has always been considered healthy as it contains beneficial vitamins and minerals as well as fructose. However, if one is insulin resistant, has pre-diabetes or type 2 diabetes, then fruit with a high sugar content, such as bananas, should be limited.

Sugar substitutes

It is important to remember that while honey and maple syrup may be less processed, they are still sugar!

Artificial sweeteners are found in diet soft drinks and many other foods. There are three different classes of sweeteners – sugar alcohols (erythritol, xylitol), artificial sweeteners (aspartame, sucralose) and natural sweeteners (stevia).

There is much debate about the merits and safety of artificial sweeteners, and they have been linked with weight gain and changes to the gut microbiome.

As mentioned previously, we have all become addicted to sweetness, so when reducing the amount of added sugar, the addition of artificial sweeteners can satisfy that urge. Our preference is for sugar alcohols and natural sweeteners, and they can be useful in the short-term while weaning yourself off sugar. However, long-term use is not advised.

Learn more

Many people ask me if they will have to go low-carb for the rest of their lives. Scan the QR code to watch Defeat Diabetes expert Dr Paul Mason and me explain why the answer isn't straightforward.

CASE STUDY | Toni Bahler

Weight loss: 10kg in two months

HbA1c: Down from 11.1 to 7

Age: 57

Summary: Toni is no stranger to the low-carb life-style; she'd successfully followed this approach for many years. After relocating to a remote town as a community midwife, however, Toni found herself so immersed in helping others that she failed to notice her old eating habits creeping back. After a routine check-up, she learnt that her HbA1c was at 11.1. It was a rude awakening.

Within two months of joining the Defeat Diabetes Program, Toni has lost 10kg, her waist-line is down 15cm, and her HbA1c is currently at 7 . . . and she's not stopping there.

Story: Many years ago, I was diagnosed with pre-diabetes with an HbA1c of 6.1. I went on a strict low-carb diet, and I got my HbA1c under 5 (no longer in the pre-diabetes range). I loved the weight-loss aspect and the general feeling of well-being, so I continued eating this way for around five years.

Amid the Covid-19 pandemic, I relocated to Broken Hill for my work and in a matter of months, I became a full-on carb addict.

In June 2021, I felt pretty ordinary. I was suffering headaches and constantly felt tired. A routine check-up returned my HbA1c at 11.1 – well over the threshold for type 2 diabetes. When the doctor put me on medication, I just felt like I'd let myself down. I really didn't want things to get worse, and I simply couldn't ignore it, so I was pleased when I happened to open an email from Low Carb Down Under, which had information about a new lifestyle program: Defeat Diabetes. I already understood the low-carb approach and had done it once before, so I decided to sign up.

I like that the program is based on science, and I love that it is Australian. I've found the program is presented in a really helpful way, and it's helped to re-educate me, and to validate what I already knew. I've watched all the Masterclasses, and often go back and watch them again! I like looking at the recipes, but to be honest, I usually keep things pretty simple, with meats and salad, steak, bacon, eggs and some cheese. I only eat one to two meals a day because I'm just not hungry. I am no longer looking for carbs.

7

Does eating fat make you fat?

'Eating fat makes you fat.' That sounds pretty logical and has been preached for the past 50 years. Consequently, we have been told specifically to reduce saturated fat (animal fats) and increase polyunsaturated fats (vegetable oils).

The only problem is that this advice is totally wrong, and one of the main reasons we have been getting fatter and sicker with each passing generation.

What are fats?

Dietary fats are a key provider of essential fats and fat-soluble vitamins. All fat-containing foods have a mixture of the three different types of fats – saturated, monounsaturated and polyunsaturated fats – but the proportions vary. It is actually impossible to eat saturated or polyunsaturated fat alone. Dairy products are the only foods with more saturated than unsaturated fat.

Saturated fat

Saturated fat is found mainly in animal products such as meat and dairy as well as certain plant foods, such as coconut and palm oil. Saturated fats are required for the absorption of the vital fat-soluble vitamins – A, E, D and K – and have been shown to raise levels of high-density lipoprotein (HDL) and promote brain health.

For many years, saturated fat has been demonised and blamed for a variety of diseases, especially heart disease. I always assumed that this was based on solid scientific evidence, but it turns out that there is really no evidence to support this position. There are now numerous studies showing that not only does saturated fat not have any negative effects on heart disease and other chronic conditions, but it may in fact have health benefits, including reducing appetite and losing weight.

Saturated fats such as butter, lard and beef tallow were used by our grandparents in cooking, but have been regrettably replaced by cheaper polyunsaturated oils. Our grandparents probably had it right!

Monounsaturated fats

Monounsaturated fats are found in many foods and are the predominant fat in some of the healthiest ingredients – avocado, olive oil, egg yolks and nuts.

Polyunsaturated fatty acids (PUFAs)

For the past 40 years, we have been encouraged to replace saturated fats (e.g. butter) with PUFAs (e.g. margarine) to the point where a significant proportion of our daily calories come from PUFAs. As previously mentioned, there is no good scientific evidence to support this switch.

There are two types of PUFAs – omega-3 and omega-6 fats. These are both essential, but we have got the proportions all wrong.

Omega-3 fatty acids are anti-inflammatory and largely beneficial to our health. Research has shown that higher levels of omega-3 are associated with a reduction in the likelihood of a heart attack, as well as having benefits for obesity and type 2 diabetes. Common foods high in omega-3 fatty acids include oily fish, fish oils, flaxseeds and oil, chia seeds and walnuts.

Omega-6 fats tend to be more inflammatory. Vegetable oils, which should more correctly be termed seed oils, are the main source of omega-6 fatty acids.

Originally used as cleaning products, these omega-6 fats are extracted from seeds, such as soybeans, corn, rapeseed and safflower, and undergo extensive processing, including bleaching, deodorising and colouring, before they are sold as healthy 'vegetable oils'. Their increased use as cheap cooking oils used in nearly all processed and junk foods means that the ratio of omega-6 to omega-3, which was approximately 1:1 a few decades ago, is now closer to 20:1. This has had disastrous health consequences.

They also tend to become oxidised or rancid during cooking, storage and processing. In the production of fast food, these industrial seed oils are repeatedly heated, resulting in more toxic by-products, such as trans fats, aldehydes and peroxides.

The other widespread use of these industrial seed oils has been in margarine, which is promoted as 'heart-healthy'. The decision to replace the natural foods of butter, lard, tallow and olive oil with chemical concoctions full of inflammatory omega-6 fats will surely go down as one of the worst decisions of our generation.

Fortunately, many people are coming to understand this and there has been a recent return to the use of butter instead of margarine.

To improve your omega-6 to omega-3 ratio, it is simply a matter of reducing the intake of seed oils, such as vegetable, soybean, soy, canola and safflower, and increasing the intake of foods high in omega-3, such as the oily fish (salmon, mackerel, tuna, sardines), walnuts, chia seeds and flaxseeds.

Which fats should we eat?

As we have seen, the advice from the past few decades to replace saturated fats with polyunsaturated fats is nonsensical.

We should:

- ▶ Eat foods high in saturated fats – meat, eggs, dairy
- ▶ Eat foods high in monounsaturated fats – olive oil, nuts, avocado
- ▶ Eat foods high in omega-3 PUFAs – oily fish, walnuts, chia seeds
- ▶ Cook with butter, coconut oil, ghee, lard, olive oil, tallow

and limit consumption of:

- ▶ Processed foods high in omega-6 polyunsaturated fats – margarine and vegetable (seed) oils, such as soybean, corn, cottonseed, safflower and rapeseed/canola oils

Learn more

You can learn more about why fat has been unfairly demonised – and why we recommend eating more! – and why seed oils like vegetable and sunflower oil are bad for you. Just scan the QR code to watch my videos.

8

How much protein?

Proteins are made up of many different amino acids – organic compounds that are essential building blocks for life – linked together, and our bodies are made up of thousands of different proteins, each with a specific function.

Proteins make up the structural components of our cells, tissues, enzymes and hormones, and are active in growth and repair.

How much protein should we eat?

The official recommended daily allowance for protein is 0.8 grams per kilogram of body weight, which equates to 56 grams of protein for a 70kg person. This is way too low for optimal health and needs to be revised.

Many people, especially older people who are

at greater risk of losing muscle mass, would benefit from a higher protein intake, somewhere around 1.2–1.5 grams per kilogram of body weight, even up to 2 grams per kilogram, per day.

Where can I get protein from?

Protein foods come from both animals and plant sources:

▶ Animal sources – red meats, pork, chicken, fish, eggs and dairy products
▶ Plant sources – grains, legumes (beans, peas and lentils), nuts, seeds and foods made from soybeans, such as tempeh and tofu

It is important to remember that the weight of the food does not equal the protein in that food. For example, a 250-gram steak does not mean 250 grams of protein.

In fact, most animal foods, including cheese, meat and eggs, are about 25 per cent protein, so that 250-gram steak is about 63 grams of protein.

Grams of protein in animal and plant sources

	Grams of protein per 100 grams
Beef	30
Chicken	31
Salmon	18
Eggs	12.6
Milk	3
Cheese	23
Greek yoghurt	4
Lentils (cooked)	9
Beans	8
Tofu	12
Almonds	21
Walnuts	15

Another advantage of eating foods containing protein is satiety. Protein (and fats) make you full, in contrast to carbohydrates, which only temporarily reduce hunger.

Learn more

To understand more about the role of protein in the diet, scan the QR code to watch the Defeat Diabetes Masterclass.

9

What should I eat?

Now it is time to look at what foods we should be eating.

What do we want to get from what we eat? Food needs to be healthy (to lower our risk of chronic disease), tasty (so we stick to our new way of eating) and affordable (so we can purchase the correct foods).

If I wanted to sum up what we should eat in one sentence, it would be:

*EAT **REAL** FOOD.*

Take inspiration from the way your grandparents ate and ditch the ultra-processed, high-sugar, high-carb foods for real foods, like:

▶ Meat
▶ Fish

- ▶ Eggs
- ▶ Dairy
- ▶ Vegetables
- ▶ Fruit
- ▶ Nuts and seeds
- ▶ Olive oil

Meat

Meat, especially red meat, has had a bad rap lately. Is that deserved?

Red meat is a nutrient-dense food and an excellent source of protein. Unlike most plants, it contains all the essential amino acids, including vitamin B12, which has to come from our food because our bodies can't synthesise it. It is also the best food source of iron, zinc and selenium.

In recent years, some observational studies have associated the consumption of red meat with various chronic diseases, such as bowel cancer. This is possibly due to the fact that meat eaters are more likely to be smokers, obese and physically inactive, as well as have a lower intake of fruit and vegetables. Cooking meat with industrial seed oils and eating it with commercial sauces can also be detrimental to one's health.

The highest level of scientific evidence has failed to confirm the link between red meat and chronic disease, though there is some evidence supporting a link between processed meats, such as hot dogs, and cancer.

There is some evidence suggesting that grass-fed meat is healthier than grain-fed, probably due to the higher omega-6 content in grain-fed meat.

Bacon has been especially demonised lately due to its saturated fat content (not as high as its monosaturated fat) and nitrate content (not that high). Bacon is probably like most other meats – it depends on how it is raised and prepared. Pigs raised on factory farms and fed grains are likely to be less healthy than free-range pigs grazing outside and eating a variety of foods. I am comfortable eating bacon purchased from my free-range butcher.

Organ meats such as liver, tongue, heart, kidneys and brain are highly nutritious, while bone broth, both homemade and commercial, contains collagen, which may have beneficial effects for skin texture, the gut and cognition. Ham, salami, sausages and luncheon meat are all low in carbs (except if breaded or sugar-glazed) and can be eaten in moderation.

Fish
Fish, in particular oily fish such as salmon, sardines, mackerel and tuna, is among the healthiest of foods due to its high omega-3 and protein content, and should ideally be eaten a couple of times a week.

Eggs
Eggs have also had a bad rap for the past few decades, due to our obsession with cholesterol levels. This is in

spite of the fact that it has been known for years that the cholesterol in the food we eat has minimal impact on our blood cholesterol levels.

Eggs are one of the most highly nutritious foods. In addition to protein, they contain healthy fats, vitamins, minerals, various antioxidants, choline, selenium and vitamin D. There does not seem to be any limit to the amount of eggs one can safely consume. Personally, I try to have a couple of eggs every day.

Dairy

Dairy is another food that has been much maligned of late, and we have been encouraged to choose low-fat dairy products. This has been another terrible mistake. If you can tolerate dairy, then full-fat dairy products provide clear benefits to bone health and cardiovascular health. Low-fat dairy contains higher levels of sugar.

However, a significant proportion of people do not tolerate dairy. Lactose intolerance is a common digestive problem, affecting 75 per cent of the world's population. It's most prevalent in Asia and South America. Those who are lactose intolerant do not have enough of the enzyme lactase, so lactose passes through the gut undigested, resulting in nausea, abdominal pain, bloating and diarrhoea.

Another group of people do not tolerate dairy products because they are sensitive to one of the milk proteins, usually the A1 protein, which they find inflammatory.

Many with lactose intolerance can digest a small amount of dairy, particularly butter, hard cheese, full-fat yoghurt and full-fat cream.

Vegetables

Vegetables are generally very healthy, being full of fibre as well as vitamins, minerals and phytonutrients. The only exception is starchy vegetables, which should be avoided by those with type 2 diabetes or pre-diabetes. These include below-the-ground vegetables, such as potatoes, parsnips and sweet potatoes.

Carb content of vegetables*

Low-carb	Medium-carb	High-carb (starchy)
Avocado	Beetroot	Corn
Asparagus	Butternut squash	Parsnips
Bok choy	Carrot	Potatoes
Broccoli	Leek	Sweet potatoes
Brussels sprouts	Peas	
Cabbage	Pumpkin	
Capsicum		
Cauliflower		
Cucumber		
Eggplant		
English spinach		
Green beans		

Low-carb	Medium-carb	High-carb (starchy)
Kale		
Lettuce		
Mushrooms		
Onion		
Radish		
Silverbeet		
Tomato		
Yellow squash		
Zucchini		

*Technically some of these are fruits

Fruits

Fruits are often lumped together with vegetables ('fruit and vegetables' are promoted as healthy and we are advised to eat at least two pieces of fruit a day). Compared to vegetables, however, fruit is not nearly as healthy. Fruit contains fibre, a few vitamins, no minerals, no essential fats and no complete protein. It does, however, contain a lot of sugar.

The fructose contained in fruit is a particular concern as it is metabolised by the liver, where excess is converted into triglycerides with the potential to lead to fatty liver, abdominal obesity and cardiovascular disease.

Not surprisingly, it is the sweeter-tasting fruits that have the highest sugar content. These fruits, which should be avoided if you have type 2 diabetes, include grapes, mangoes, pineapple, watermelon and bananas. Dried fruit is also high in sugar.

My favourite fruits are berries, especially strawberries, raspberries and blackberries – blueberries are a bit higher in sugar content and carbohydrates.

Here is a list of fruits divided into sugar content:

Sugar content of fruits

Low-sugar	Medium-sugar	High-sugar
Apricot	Apple	Banana
Blackberries	Cherries	Dates
Blueberries	Fig	Grapes
Grapefruit	Honeydew melon	Mango
Kiwifruit	Nectarine	Pineapple
Lemon	Orange	Prunes
Lime	Passionfruit	Raisins
Mandarin	Peach	Watermelon
Raspberries	Pear	
Rhubarb	Plum	
Strawberries	Rockmelon	
	Tangerine	

Even more damaging are fruit juice, fruit drinks and fruit smoothies. In these, all the fibre and much of the goodness has been removed, leaving only sugar and water.

I do have one favourite fruit, although many people don't realise it is a fruit: avocados are full of healthy fats and are arguably the most nutritious fruit around.

Nuts and seeds

Nuts are high in healthy fats, vitamin E, magnesium, selenium and antioxidants known as polyphenols, all while being low in carbs. Seeds are good sources of protein, minerals, zinc and other nutrients. There is a large variety of nuts and seeds, which can be eaten in many different ways. The healthiest way to eat nuts is raw or oven-roasted below 175°C. Make sure you avoid nuts roasted in vegetable (seed) oils.

My favourite nuts are macadamias, almonds, hazelnuts, walnuts and Brazil nuts, and my favourite seeds are sunflower, pumpkin, sesame, chia, hemp and flax.

Olive oil

Olive oil is regarded as a very healthy food due to its high monounsaturated fat content. It also contains large amounts of the powerful antioxidants polyphenols. It can oxidise when heated above 180°C, so use it for salad dressings, or drizzle it over vegetables, meats or fish that have already been cooked.

Salt

Salt is another food that has been demonised for the last few decades.

'Salt is bad for you.'

'You must reduce your salt intake.'

As with most things nutrition-related, it's not that simple. Evidence shows that both a very high and a very low intake of salt is detrimental. On the current highly processed diet common among Australians, excessive salt is more likely, and the source of that salt is all the processed food because, along with sugar and grains, many processed foods contain added salt.

However, when you eliminate processed food from your diet and eat a diet consisting of real food, you are quite likely to be too low in your salt intake. That is thought to be the cause of the so-called 'keto flu', which affects people who switch to a very low-carbohydrate diet with no processed food in the first few weeks of their new way of eating.

If you continue to eat a diet full of real food and avoid highly salted processed food, you will need to continue adding salt to your food to keep up sufficient salt (sodium) to perform its vital functions. Remember: salt is essential for every cell in the body.

How often should you eat?

Wild animals never seem to have a problem with their weight, even if there is an abundance of food. This is because, on a natural diet, their appetites are appropriately regulated. We see the reverse of this in newspaper stories about fat zoo animals and obese pets, where factors such as unnaturally sugary modern fruit- and grain-based foods are at play.

We humans are no different. Left to the whims of our appetite on a diet of sugary, carbohydrate-rich processed food, we will reliably gain weight. However, if we are able to forgo processed foods and focus on nutrient-dense real food, our appetites often decrease without any conscious awareness. This can lead to significant weight loss without hunger.

Of course, the key is to only eat when we are truly hungry. This means that we must disabuse ourselves of the notion that we need to eat several times per day, and stop eating to the clock. Our meals need to be nourishing enough, and of sufficient size, to fill us up.

This also means making sure there is both enough protein and fat, and not too much carbohydrates. People who are afraid of fat end up consuming things like salads, which are really not very filling, and lead to hunger within a few hours.

You should also be mindful to only eat when you are hungry, not merely to satisfy cravings, such as for sweet foods. You can often tell the difference by asking what it is you feel like. If you would not eat healthy low-carb food like an omelette, some cheese or lamb chops, chances are you are not really hungry.

Following these principles, many people end up comfortably eating twice a day, even without snacks.

Remember: only eat when you are *truly* hungry.

CASE STUDY | David Velleley

Weight loss: 30kg

HbA1c: 20 down to 5 (no longer in type 2 diabetes range)

Summary: When David was diagnosed with type 2 diabetes, he was told there was no cure. Distraught but refusing to accept this fate, he went on a fact-finding mission and discovered the Defeat Diabetes Program. Within weeks, David was seeing results that astonished his GP. One year on, he's 30kg lighter, his diabetes is in remission, and he's off his medication entirely.

Story: I've always been in reasonably good shape and prioritised my fitness. But when the pandemic hit, I craved sweet food, drank more beer than usual and gradually (and inevitably) put on weight.

When my cravings worsened and I was urinating more frequently, I thought that I must have type 2 diabetes, or at least be at risk. My father had his leg amputated from diabetes-related complications and I knew if I turned a blind eye and didn't act, I, too, would get to the point where I could die.

After a visit to my GP, my worst fears were confirmed. I had developed type 2 diabetes. Even though I was half-expecting it, I was devastated.

My GP told me it was a progressive and

irreversible condition, and immediately put me on metformin. She said the only way I could manage it was with more and more insulin as the disease worsened. But I didn't want to believe it, so I started doing my research. That's when I came discovered the Defeat Diabetes Program.

Within weeks of following the meal plans, my GP sent a text message, asking me to call her urgently. I thought it was going to be bad news, but she was astounded because my lipids had dropped from dangerous levels to healthy in just a few weeks. She couldn't believe her eyes!

When I started the program, I thought it couldn't be true that I could improve my condition by eating cream and fatty foods. But it really works! I feel healthier than I've ever been in my life.

One year on, I'm 30kg lighter, my type 2 diabetes is in remission and I'm entirely off my medication. My eyesight is improving, I no longer have 'word vomit', I sleep better, and all my sugar cravings are gone. Luckily for my wife (and me), she reports that I no longer snore! The best part is my doctor says I'll live longer.

The program has taught me everything I need to improve my blood glucose control. I've got the confidence to get more creative in the kitchen, enjoying simple creations like a scotch fillet with onions, mushrooms, spinach and broccoli cooked in butter or scrambled eggs with salmon and avocado, and blueberries with full-fat cream for dessert.

My advice for anyone considering signing up for Defeat Diabetes is just to give it a go. It works! In fact, it's life-changing.

10

Red, amber and green foods

Evidence shows a low-carb approach can help send pre-diabetes and type 2 diabetes into remission. Follow this handy food guide to better manage your blood sugars and find improved health.

Eat plenty of 'green' foods

Red meat	Beef Lamb	Pork Organ meats
Cured meat	Bacon Biltong Jerky	Parma ham Prosciutto Salami
Poultry	Chicken Duck	Turkey
Fish	All fish	All shellfish

Eggs		
Vegetables	Asparagus	Kale
	Broccoli	Leek
	Brussels sprouts	Lettuce
	Cabbage	Mushroom
	Capsicum	Onion
	Cauliflower	Olives
	Cucumber	Spinach
	Green beans	Zucchini
Fruit	Avocado	Raspberries
	Blackberries	Strawberries
Fats and oils	Butter	Goose fat
	Ghee (clarified butter)	Coconut oil
		Olive oil
	Tallow (beef fat)	Avocado
	Duck fat	Macadamia oil
	Lard (pork fat)	(dressings only)
Condiments	Vegemite	Vinegars
Dairy (avoid reduced-fat dairy)	Cream	Full-fat Greek yoghurt
	Sour cream	Full-fat milk
	All cheeses	Dark chocolate
	Cream cheese	(85%+ cocoa)
Drinks	Water	Bone broth
	Black coffee	Soda water
	Tea	Mineral water

Eat some 'amber' foods

Starchy vegetables	Beetroot Butternut squash Carrot	Peas Pumpkin
Fruit	Apple Apricot Blueberries Kiwifruit Lemon Lime Orange	Peach Pear Plum Rockmelon Tomatoes Watermelon
Nuts and seeds	Almonds Brazil nuts Cashews Chia seeds Flaxseeds Hazelnuts Linseed	Macadamias Peanuts Pistachios Pumpkin seeds Sesame seeds Sunflower seeds Walnuts
Flours	Almond flour	Coconut flour
Condiments	Barbecue sauce (low-sugar) Dijon mustard Seeded mustard	Tabasco Tamari Tomato sauce (low-sugar)
Artificial sweeteners (natural only)	Erythritol Monk fruit	Stevia Xylitol
Alcohol	Dry wines Low-carb beer	White spirits (gin, vodka)

Eat few 'red' foods

Sugar, fast food, processed food (not limited to)	Biscuits Cakes Chocolate Crisps Fruit yoghurt	Ice cream Lollies Muesli bars Pastries Sauces
Processed meats	Highly processed sausages	Luncheon meats
Fruit	Banana Dried fruit Grapes	Mango Pineapple
Starches and cereals	Barley Bread Breakfast cereals Buckwheat Corn Couscous Crackers Crumpets Gnocchi Millet Muesli Muffins Noodles	Oats Pasta Potato chips Potatoes Polenta Quinoa Rice Rice cakes Rye Sorghum Sweet potato Wheat

Legumes	Alfalfa
	Beans (soybeans,
	  navy, mung,
	  broad/fava, lima,
	  lupins, kidney and
	  borlotti)
	Carob
		Chickpeas
		Clover
		Lentils
		Mesquite
		Peas (all types)
		Tamarind

Fats and oils	'Butter' spreads Margarine	Vegetable/seed oils (canola, sunflower, safflower, cottonseed, rapeseed, soybean, corn)
Artificial sweeteners	Diet drinks Equal	Splenda Sucaryl
Condiments	Barbecue sauce Honey Jam Maple syrup	Marmalade Sweet chilli sauce Tomato sauce
Drinks	Cordials Energy drinks Flavoured milks Fruit juices	Nut milks Soft drinks Sports drinks
Alcohol	Beer Cider Dessert wines	Liqueurs Sugary mixers (tonic, cola, Red Bull)

11

What should I avoid eating ... and what can I eat instead?

Real foods are nutrient-dense and good for your health.

Processed foods, on the other hand, are nutrient-hollow and are full of sugar, unhealthy fats, usually in the form of vegetable (seed) oils, synthetic emulsifiers, which have a negative effect on gut health, and artificial flavourings and additives.

'Processed' covers all foods that are pre-boxed or in wrappers, and includes processed grains:

- ▶ Breakfast cereals and cereal bars
- ▶ Baked goods, including cakes, biscuits and crackers
- ▶ Snacks, including but not limited to popcorn, corn chips and potato chips
- ▶ Sugar-sweetened beverages, diet drinks and fruit juice
- ▶ Margarines, jams and sugary spreads

- ▶ Pasta and rice
- ▶ Flavoured yoghurts
- ▶ Breads and grains
- ▶ Commercial sauces
- ▶ Instant soups
- ▶ Chicken nuggets and fish fingers
- ▶ Processed meats, such as sausages and hamburgers
- ▶ Many ready-to-heat meals, such as pies and pizzas
- ▶ Chocolate and other confectionery
- ▶ Ice cream and other sugary desserts

It is best to avoid processed foods as much as possible. Try to stay on the periphery of the supermarket, where most of the healthy foods (meat, fish, dairy, fruit and vegetables) are placed, and avoid the middle aisles with the packaged processed foods.

'But what if I love pizza, pasta, rice and/or bread?' I hear you ask.

Well, there are great alternatives.

Processed food	Healthy alternative
Pasta noodles	Zucchini noodles (see Zucchini Carbonara on page 238)
Pizza	'Fat head', cauliflower pizza or Margherita Pizza (page 235)

Processed food	Healthy alternative
Rice	Low-Carb Cauliflower Fried Rice (page 242)
Packaged breakfast cereal	Homemade nuts and seeds muesli (see Dr Brukner's Oat-free Muesli on page 166)
Packaged bread	Commercial low-carb breads or homemade breads (see Three-seed Bread on page 182)
Commercial sauces/mayonnaise	Reduced sugar or homemade sauces/mayonnaise (see Healthy Mayonnaise on page 252 and Homemade Tomato Sauce on page 254)
Milk chocolate	Dark chocolate (85%+ cocoa)

CASE STUDY | Shane Dobson

Weight loss: 26kg in eight months

HbA1c: Down 7.6 to 5.3 (no longer in type 2 diabetes range)

Age: 67

Summary: After being diagnosed with type 2 diabetes 15 years ago, living with persistently high blood sugar became the norm for Shane, a retiree from Gippsland. After a further diagnosis of Parkinson's disease, then learning he had fatty liver disease and his highest HbA1c in a long time, he knew things were heading in the wrong direction.

Since adopting a low-carb way of eating, Shane has lost 26kg and now prioritises his diet and daily exercise. As a result, his HbA1c has dropped and he's reduced his medications, and the benefits don't stop there.

Story: I've lived with type 2 diabetes for 15 years. Before discovering Defeat Diabetes, I thought I ate reasonably well. However, in hindsight, I was solely focused on avoiding sugar, and didn't think about the carbohydrates I was eating. I'd eat a bowl of pasta or potatoes for dinner most evenings and believed I was doing the right thing by eating starchy carbs. But now I know that they contributed to my high blood sugar levels.

In May 2021, my HbA1c was 7.6 – the highest in quite a while. I also had signs of fatty liver and, two years prior, I'd been diagnosed with Parkinson's disease. I knew if I wanted to be around for a while longer, I had to try to improve my health.

I saw an advertisement on TV about Defeat Diabetes, so I joined the program and started watching the videos and reading the articles. As I went through the program, it all began to make sense. It turned everything I knew about nutrition upside down, and I was amazed to learn that even a bowl of pasta was doing as much harm as a teaspoon of sugar.

After eight months, I've lost 26kg (on average about 1.2kg a week), and my wife, Betty, has lost over 10kg by adopting this way of eating with me.

As well as the weight loss, my blood pressure has improved, I've reduced my medications, my energy levels have increased and the tremor in my left hand from Parkinson's disease has reduced. My GP couldn't believe my results. After seeing what it's done for me in such a short time, he's supportive of the low-carb approach.

I follow the principles of the program rather than following a super strict diet. Still, I'm constantly referring back to the content in the program, in particular the Traffic Light Guide, which outlines the foods that I can enjoy (and those that I need to limit) on a low-carb diet. I've printed it out and stuck it to our fridge to help plan the weekly shopping.

I've learnt to reduce my portion sizes and curb cravings (although I still enjoy a sneaky meat pie from time to time). I've replaced pasta and potatoes with omelettes, meats, salad and cauliflower mash.

My wife and I prioritise exercise, walking 5–6km daily. We love our newfound routine so much that we're disappointed if we don't get to go on our walk when it's a rainy day!

The results will be there if you're committed to learning how to manage type 2 diabetes through diet. It's simple, not complicated. You're not counting calories, just eating sensibly. It just makes sense.

12

What should I drink?

You won't be surprised to hear that there's no question that water is the healthiest drink and, most often, tap water will do the trick. If you are concerned about the quality of your tap water, it may be an idea to install a filter or buy a filter jug.

Unlimited drinks are:

▶ Water
▶ Tea
▶ Coffee
▶ Bone broth and bouillon

Now that we're clear on what you can drink, let's move on to what to avoid:

▶ Carbonated soft drinks – colas, lemonade (see page 74 for more on why diet soft drinks aren't a good substitute)

- ▶ Energy drinks and 'isotonic' sports drinks – Gatorade, Powerade
- ▶ Vitamin water and other commercial flavoured waters
- ▶ Fruit juices and smoothies
- ▶ Cordials
- ▶ Iced teas
- ▶ Flavoured milk

The following drinks may be suitable in limited servings, if you can tolerate small amounts of sugar:

- ▶ Milk
- ▶ Coconut water
- ▶ Vegetable juices
- ▶ Homemade flavoured mineral water (either with slices of fruit and fresh herbs added, or infused with food-grade essential oils, to give a fruity scent)
- ▶ Kombucha

What about alcohol?

The World Health Organization suggests that the ideal amount of alcohol for your health is zero. However, if you are going to have a drink, limit yourself to one to two drinks, two to three times a week.

Alcohol has been shown to slow down fat-burning so think carefully before you indulge.

What about the carbohydrate content of alcoholic drinks?

Wines including dry white, red and champagne are relatively low in carbs. Sweeter wines are, not surprisingly, higher.

Spirits such as gin, brandy, whiskey and vodka are high in alcohol content but low in carbs. Be careful of high-carb mixers such as cola, tonic, Red Bull and orange juice.

Liqueurs such as Baileys and Kahlua are high in carbs and best avoided.

	Higher carb	Lower carb
Wine	Sweet white and red wines, dessert wines, mulled wines	Dry red and white, champagne
Spirits & mixed drinks	Mixers – cola, tonic, Red Bull, juices	Gin, brandy, whiskey, tequila, vodka Soda, diet tonic
Liqueurs	Baileys, Kahlua, Amaretto	

	Higher carb	Lower carb
Coolers, Alcopops	Most (wine coolers, Smirnoff Ice, Bacardi Breezer, etc.)	
Cocktails	Most (margarita, white Russian, daiquiri, cosmopolitan, pina colada)	Dry martinis
Beers* and ciders	Most	Some low-carb beers*

*See below

Most beers are high in carb content (around 10–15g per 355ml bottle) but there are an increasing number of low-carb (less than 5g carbs per 355ml bottle) beers coming on to the market. There is even a growing number of options that claim to have zero carbs.

Low-carb beers (less than 5g carbs per 355ml bottle)

	Carbs (grams per 355ml)
Burleigh Big Head	0
Better Beer	0
Pure Blonde Ultra Low-Carb	1.7
Hahn Super Dry	2.2
Hahn Super Dry 3.5	2.5

	Carbs (grams per 355ml)
Steersman Blonde	2.6
XXXX Summer Bright Lager	2.7
Skinny Lager	3.0
Hahn Super Dry Premium	3.0
Coopers Dry	3.3
Coopers Clear	3.6
Iron Jack Crisp Australian lager	3.7
Pure Blonde Premium Mid	3.9
Iron Jack Full Strength lager	4.2
Hahn Ultra Crisp	4.5

13

And there's more ...

While the focus of this book is on the importance of a low-carbohydrate eating pattern to improve blood glucose control, there are some other important contributors both to improved general health and glucose control: exercise, sleep, stress and sun.

Exercise

There is substantial evidence that exercise can provide benefits for more than 30 different chronic diseases, including type 2 diabetes. Regular exercise has been shown to improve blood glucose control, with studies showing reductions of 0.5 per cent to 0.7 per cent in HbA1c levels, indicating a significant improvement in blood glucose.

Exercise can also play a role in weight loss, but not nearly as significant as diet. It's true what they say, you can't outrun a bad diet!

So what type of exercise?

The best exercise to do is the one that you will maintain, therefore it is important to find one that you enjoy. That is very much up to the individual. Some like running, others swimming or cycling. Some prefer to play competitive sport such as tennis, other get their exercise on the golf course. Some like to work out in groups such as at a gym or leisure centre, others enjoy solitude while listening to music or a podcast.

And how much?

The Australian Government's *Physical Activity and Sedentary Behaviour Guidelines (2014)* recommend that adult Australians aged 18–64:

- ▶ Be active on most, preferably all, days
- ▶ Accumulate 150–300 minutes of moderately intense physical activity or 75–150 minutes of vigorously intense physical activity, or a combination of the two, each week. For example, in one week, you might do three one-hour moderate sessions or two intense sessions of 45 minutes each.

- ▶ Do muscle-strengthening activities for at least two of your physical activity sessions each week. This could be lifting weights at the gym, or dancing, cycling, yoga or Pilates.
- ▶ Break up any periods of sitting, ideally at least every 30 minutes

That seems like pretty good advice. One point that often gets missed, though, is resistance exercise.

As we get older, we naturally lose muscle strength. The average person loses muscle mass initially at around eight per cent per decade. However, this accelerates to 15 per cent after the age of 70, with a heightened risk of physical decline that can impair mobility, with potentially disastrous effects on one's future health. So the sooner you get in the resistance exercise habit, the better! There is even evidence that resistance exercise improves insulin sensitivity in those with type 2 diabetes.

Some people think resistance exercise equals pumping massive amounts of iron in a fancy gym surrounded by bodybuilders and accompanied by loud music! None of that is necessary, though.

There are many simple exercises you can do at home, including squats, push-ups, star jumps and burpees. Doing a series of home exercises for 15–20 minutes two or three times a week is sufficient. My favourite exercise is the single leg squat, which is great for balance as well. You can do it anywhere at any time!

You can also increase the amount of exercise you do in your everyday activities, such as walking (especially up and down stairs), housekeeping, gardening, carrying shopping bags etc.

Sleep

Poor-quality sleep has a detrimental effect on blood glucose control. Just one night of sleep deprivation can lead to disruptions in insulin sensitivity similar to six months of unhealthy eating. One study followed 1455 adults for six years and found that fasting glucose levels were significantly higher in those who slept less than six hours a night.

How much sleep do we need? Once again, it varies from individual to individual. Authorities have traditionally recommended seven to nine hours a night. When we get less than seven hours of sleep, we don't perform at our best. When we habitually get less than six hours sleep a night, our risk of health problems increases.

The quality of sleep, such as reduced length, interrupted or a lack of deep sleep, is just as important as the total length.

Here are some things you can do to help ensure a good night's sleep:

During the day
- ▶ Get natural sunlight
- ▶ Make your bed
- ▶ Exercise, preferably outdoors

In the evening
- ▶ Avoid excess alcohol
- ▶ Eat a light dinner and stop eating three hours before bedtime
- ▶ Curtail the caffeine
- ▶ Have a calming tea

Before you go to bed
- ▶ Stick to a regular schedule
- ▶ No bright artificial lights or TV in the bedroom
- ▶ Avoid using your phone, tablet or laptop in bed
- ▶ Don't drink any fluids within two hours of going to bed
- ▶ Avoid before-bed snacks, particularly grains, sugars and caffeinated drinks
- ▶ Try to unwind mentally

During the night
- ▶ Keep the temperature in your bedroom no higher than 21°C
- ▶ Consider separate bedrooms if your partner disturbs you
- ▶ Keep it dark

Stress

Stress can be a major barrier to effective glucose control. Stress hormones, including cortisol, directly affect glucose levels. When you are stressed, your body releases adrenaline and cortisol into your bloodstream, causing your blood glucose levels to rise.

Many techniques can be utilised to reduce stress. Examples are improved sleep, regular physical activity, meditation, mindfulness, yoga, healthy eating and music, and just taking time to replenish yourself a little bit each day. Connecting with nature can also be calming and grounding.

Social connectedness is also important, and time spent on relationships with family and friends is essential, but often undervalued.

Sun

Given our climate, no Australian should ever be vitamin D deficient, and yet we are seeing more and more deficiencies. Australia has gone from a nation of sun worshippers to a country that fears and avoids the sun. My generation spent far too much time baking in the hot sun when we were children. We regularly got sunburnt and, not surprisingly, started developing skin cancers at a great rate.

As a result of an extremely effective campaign from the Cancer Council (slip, slop, slap – surely one of the cleverest slogans ever), the current generation of children studiously avoid the rays of the sun by minimising exposure to direct sunlight, or when exposed, ensure protection from clothing or SPF-15 sunscreen.

The success of this campaign has inadvertently led to deficiencies of vitamin D, a hormone produced by the skin on exposure to sunlight and one that plays a vital role in many body processes. Vitamin D has been shown to have a positive effect on the following conditions:

- ▶ All-cause mortality
- ▶ Bone health
- ▶ Falls in the elderly, due to improved muscle strength and balance
- ▶ Colorectal and breast cancer
- ▶ Age-related macular degeneration
- ▶ Depression
- ▶ Dementia, including Alzheimer's disease
- ▶ Parkinson's disease
- ▶ Premature birth

People with type 2 diabetes have lower vitamin D levels, and all-cause mortality is higher for those in this group with the lowest vitamin D levels. Vitamin D deficiency has also been associated with poor outcomes from Covid-19 infections. You can get vitamin D from your diet through oily fish, eggs, mushrooms, milk, beef liver and cod liver oil, or from supplements, but exposure to sunlight is by far the most effective means of increasing your vitamin D. I would suggest regular (daily, if possible) exposure to 20 minutes of sun, avoiding the intense heat and certainly avoiding getting burnt.

CASE STUDY | Neil Manuel

Weight loss: 16kg in 16 months

HbA1c: Down from 12.2 to 5.3 (no longer in type 2 diabetes range)

Age: 55

Summary: Neil Manuel, a 55-year-old seemingly healthy rural farmer, went for a routine check-up, thinking he'd get the all-clear for a few more years. Instead, he learnt he had type 2 diabetes and all the markers of metabolic syndrome. Since starting the Defeat Diabetes Program, he's lost 16kg in 16 months and his HbA1c has dropped from 12.2 to 5.3. Best of all, he's found a welcoming community that has given him a new zest for life and inspired him to help others around Australia.

Story: As a rural farmer, I have a pretty active job, often sheering up to 600 sheep daily! I'd never really had any health issues, didn't consider myself overweight and, like many men my age, I hadn't visited the doctors in years.

For peace of mind, my father-in-law (a man who likes to keep up-to-date with his yearly health checks) urged me to go for a long overdue health check-up. I thought it would be a simple routine visit; I couldn't have been more wrong.

I had no idea what an HbA1c was, but when the doctor said mine was shockingly high (12.2) and diagnosed me with type 2 diabetes and metabolic disease, it sent shockwaves through me.

I'd noticed all the symptoms but had just put them down to the natural ageing process: lethargy, tiredness, lack of energy, worsening eyesight, pins and needles in my feet, frequent urination and increased thirst. I thought it was all normal, but now I know it's not.

After the clinic visit, I searched for information on type 2 diabetes. Of course, the first port of call was Google, where I furiously tried to find information about my condition. A quick search for 'the best foods for type 2 diabetes' told me blueberries were good. I have to laugh about this now, but at the time, acting out of pure shock and desperation, I downed a few punnets, thinking it might instantly cure me!

Taking a more science-based approach led me to the Defeat Diabetes Program. I was a little sceptical at first, because the program suggested that by focusing on eating protein and healthy fat, I would want to eat less. I thought there was NO WAY it would work for me, because I've always been a big eater. No one will beat me in an eating competition!

But now I eat two meals a day; I couldn't

possibly fit in breakfast. I eat a third of what I used to eat, and I'm never hungry.

Better yet, my health markers have improved. My HbA1c is down to 5.3, meaning I've put my type 2 diabetes into remission! I have so much energy and I sleep solidly through the night (something I used to struggle with).

And while weight loss wasn't my motivation, I've also lost around 16kg without trying. My girl-friend reckons I'm too skinny now!

In some ways, I feel so cheated by the dietary guidelines. I can see so many flaws in the system. I used to think I ate pretty well – I even had a juicer and would make 'healthy' juices every day – but I know now that's what got me here.

I now spend every waking moment educating myself on nutrition, and I am even part of some men's health initiatives in my community. I plan to retire in five years and travel around Australia, educating people in rural communities about diet. I had no idea just how much Defeat Diabetes would change my life. I'm so grateful for all that I've learnt and incredibly thankful for people like Dr Peter Brukner and Dr Paul Mason for creating the Defeat Diabetes Program to help educate people on nutrition.

If you're thinking about this lifestyle, I reckon the key to getting better is educating yourself.

If you are open to making some simple lifestyle changes, you won't regret it. If a simple farmer can do it, then so can you!

14

FAQs and mythbusters

1. Low-carb diets work, but are not sustainable long-term

Low-carb diets are sustainable in the long-term because eating plenty of healthy fats and proteins means you are not hungry. Hunger is the main reason other diets are not sustainable.

2. Most of the weight lost on low-carb diets comes from water weight

When you start a low-carb diet and lower your insulin levels, water and salt are lost from the kidneys. However, the body rapidly adapts and subsequent weight loss is due to loss of body fat.

3. A low-carb diet will cause clogged arteries and heart attacks because it is too high in saturated fat

It has been shown in numerous scientific studies that

saturated fat from animal sources such as dairy, meat and eggs has no correlation with atherosclerosis and heart disease. This is a long-standing myth with no evidence to support it.

4. The brain needs carbs to function properly
The brain needs a small amount of glucose, which can be produced from fats and proteins by a process known as gluconeogenesis. The brain functions very well using fats, in the form of ketone bodies, as its main fuel source.

5. Dr Atkins died from heart disease
This is a commonly stated myth. Atkins died from a brain injury following a fall on ice.

6. Ketosis is dangerous and damages the kidneys
There is no evidence of kidney dysfunction on a ketogenic diet. Persistently elevated blood sugar levels damage the kidneys, so maintaining blood glucose levels within normal range on a low-carb diet can help prevent kidney disease.

7. There's not enough fibre to feed my microbiome
Low-carb diets can be quite high in fibre due to the increased ingestion of vegetables, nuts and seeds.

8. Low-carb diets suck calcium from your bones

There is no evidence that low-carb diets remove calcium from bones. In fact, low-carb diets have been shown to improve bone density in those with osteoporosis.

9. Eating meat is bad for the environment

The debate between meat vs plant diets and their impact on the environment fails to recognise the complexity of food systems. Industrialised agriculture (both plant crops and animal feedlots) is harmful to the land, soil, water and climate. Sustainable farming practices that renew soils and tackle climate change include regenerative farming and pasture-fed animals.

10. I need to eat carbs to manage my diabetes

Diabetes is a disease of carbohydrate intolerance, so controlling carbs will help to bring blood glucose levels under control. Low-carb diets have been proven to be effective in managing diabetes.

11. You need carbs for energy

The human body has two potential fuel sources for energy – carbs and fats. The body is capable of using either as its primary source.

12. Low-carb diets cause nutrient deficiencies

With a focus on real foods such as meat, fish, eggs, dairy, vegetables, nuts and seeds, your diet will be nutrient-dense. In contrast, diets full of empty calories such as junk foods, processed foods and refined grains are more likely to be nutrient-deficient.

13. Low-carb diets can lead to depression

Low-carb diets have not been shown to be associated with depression. On the contrary, there has been some interesting research from Deakin University showing improvements in depression and anxiety from a real food diet.

14. Low-carb could cause ketoacidosis

The levels of ketones associated with a low-carb or ketogenic diet are well below the levels associated with ketoacidosis. The only exception is in those patients taking SGLT2 inhibitors, which should be discontinued when commencing a low-carb diet.

15. Low-carb is too expensive

Like any diet, it is possible to select budget-friendly options. Additionally, hunger comes under control with this way of eating, and many people find themselves eating fewer snacks, eating two instead of three meals a day and eliminating discretionary food purchases, such as cake and confectionery.

16. Low-carb is bad for athletes

Many athletes, especially endurance athletes, have

switched from the traditional high-carb diet to a low-carb, high-fat diet. Fat is a very effective fuel and we all have plenty of it. You don't have to re-fuel as often, you recover better and you don't suffer the negative effects on your health from high carbohydrate intake.

17. A low-carb diet has way too much protein in it
Low-carb diets are not high-protein diets. Recommended protein intake is in line with other types of diets.

18. It doesn't matter if you eat low-carb or low-fat, the only thing that matters is calories in, calories out
While calories do matter, they are not the only factors affecting weight, and we advise against calorie counting. The hormonal response, in particular insulin, to different foods is just as important. Low-carb diets reduce the secretion of insulin.

19. Low-carb will harm your liver
Low-carb diet will improve your liver function and can reverse the condition known as non-alcoholic fatty liver disease (NAFLD).

20. Low-carb will give you gout
Low-carb diets have been shown to improve the symptoms associated with gout. Excess sugar intake is thought to be a major cause of gout.

15

My weekly meal plans and recipes

Since commencing my low-carb eating habit, I have definitely been less hungry and gone from eating three meals and three snacks a day to often eating only two meals a day. Rather than sticking rigidly to a set number of meals, one should eat when hungry. If you're not hungry, then you don't need to eat.

Having said that, let's go with a plan for three meals a day, with the occasional snack. I've included two weekly meal plans on pages 160–163.

Breakfast

A standard breakfast consists of some combination of cereal with low-fat milk, low-fat fruit yoghurt, fruit juice, toast with margarine and jam/honey/Vegemite, finished off with tea or coffee. Sound familiar? Well, congratulations! You have just exceeded your recommended daily intake of sugar – and you haven't even left home.

Instead, try a simple healthy breakfast of full-fat yoghurt, nuts, seeds and berries. Or make a cooked breakfast with some combination of eggs, bacon, mushrooms, tomatoes, spinach and avocado. Best to avoid toast, except for the occasional piece of sourdough, maybe under the smashed avocado! For Breakfast recipes, see pages 164–183.

Lunch

Traditional lunches usually revolve around bread or similar products. I try and avoid them. If I haven't already had some eggs, I will go with an egg-based meal, such as an omelette and include some vegetables, like capsicum, tomato or mushrooms. Salads, cold meats, soups or last night's leftovers are my favourites, though you should avoid any sugary dressings or croutons. For Lunch recipes, see pages 184–209.

Dinner

Dinner is pretty easy: meat or fish and plenty of vegetables or salad. No need to trim the fat off the meat, and barbecue, grill or pan-fry the meat in butter. Vegetables should be green (beans, broccoli, spinach etc.) and coloured (capsicum, cauliflower etc.). Avoid the starchy ones, such as potatoes – and that means chips as well; the combination of potatoes cooked in vegetable oil is particularly unhealthy! For Dinner recipes, see pages 210–251.

If I want dessert, berries and full-fat cream or yoghurt, or maybe a couple of squares of dark (85%+) chocolate, finish off the meal nicely.

Snacks

I don't tend to need snacks on a low-carb diet, but if I do a handful of nuts or a piece of cheese are my favourites. Other options are a boiled egg, some biltong, or some chopped veggies (zucchini, celery) with dips such as hummus, guacamole or cream cheese.

My favourite meal plans

Week One

	Sunday	Monday	Tuesday
Breakfast	Bacon, Eggs and Veg (page 164)	Dr Brukner's Oat-free Muesli (page 166)	Yoghurt, Nuts and Raspberries (page 168)
Lunch	Thai Beef Salad (page 184)	Mish-Mash Hash (page 186)	Super Simple Salmon Omelette (page 188)
Dinner	Saucy Moroccan Lamb (page 210)	Prawn Pad Thai (page 213)	One-Pan Creamy Chicken and Mushroom (page 215)

Wednesday	Thursday	Friday	Saturday
Dr Brukner's Oat-free Muesli (page 166)	Easy Crêpes (page 169)	Dr Brukner's Oat-free Muesli (page 166)	Zucchini and Feta Fritters (page 171)
Easy Ham and Veggie Wraps (page 190)	Dr Brukner's Bacon and Avocado Salad (page 192)	Chicken and Green Veg Soup (page 194)	Mediterranean Eggs and Chorizo in a Pan (page 196)
Chinese Beef and Broccoli (page 217)	Cheesy Asparagus and Spinach Tart (page 219)	Silky Salmon Curry (page 222)	Pork Schnittys with Buttery Cabbage (page 224)

Week Two

	Sunday	Monday	Tuesday
Breakfast	Raspberry Chia Pots (page 173)	Zucchini, Olive and Feta Bread (page 174)	'Noatmeal' Overnight Oats (page 176)
Lunch	Rainbow Frittata Slice (page 198)	Simple Ploughman's Platter (page 200)	Sesame Salmon Skewers (page 201)
Dinner	Ultimate Low-Carb Lasagne (page 226)	Fried Salmon with Green Beans and Pumpkin (page 229)	Steak and Baby Potato (page 231)

Wednesday	Thursday	Friday	Saturday
Zucchini, Olive and Feta Bread (page 174)	Power Brekkie (page 177)	Zucchini, Olive and Feta Bread (page 174)	Scrambled Eggs with Smoked Salmon and Avocado (page 178)
15-Minute Mexican Burrito Bowl (page 203)	Barbecue Chicken Salad (page 205)	Dukkah Fish Wraps (page 206)	Simple Grilled Lamb with Greek Salad (page 208)
Easy Sausage Tray Bake (page 233)	Margherita Pizza (page 235)	Zucchini Carbonara (page 238)	Quick Chicken Tikka Masala (page 240)

My favourite recipes

Breakfast

Bacon, Eggs and Veg

We've replaced the toast with nutritious and tasty veggies in this classic dish of bacon and eggs. Swap the mushroom or asparagus for any other veg you have on hand or happen to love. Other combos include cherry tomatoes, baby spinach and avocado.

Serves: 1 | **Cook:** 10 minutes

2 tbsp butter
2 bacon rashers
½ cup sliced button mushrooms
4 spears asparagus, woody ends trimmed
2 large free-range eggs
salt and pepper

1. Melt the butter in a large frying pan over medium heat. Add the bacon and fry until crispy. Using a slotted spoon, remove the bacon from the pan and set aside on a serving plate. Leave the residual fat in the pan.
2. Add the mushroom and asparagus to one side of the pan, crack in the eggs, and season with salt.

▶

Cook the vegetables for 3–4 minutes, until the mushroom is golden and the asparagus is tender, and fry the eggs to your liking, ensuring that the whites are set.

3. Transfer the vegetables and fried eggs to the serving plate with the bacon and season with salt and pepper to taste.

Protein	Fat	Net carbs	Fibre
36.3 grams per serve	**42.7** grams per serve	**1.8** grams per serve	**2.0** grams per serve

Dr Brukner's Oat-free Muesli

Make up a batch of Dr Brukner's low-carb muesli and you've got a healthy, no-cook breakfast or snack on standby. The cinnamon adds a natural sweetness that kids also love. If you don't have all the ingredients in your pantry, don't stress! You can easily make this muesli with whatever you have to hand, so feel free to experiment. This is best served with unsweetened thick Greek-style yoghurt and fresh berries.

Serves: 10 | **Prep:** 10 minutes

1 cup almonds, coarsely chopped
½ cup macadamia nuts, coarsely chopped
½ cup walnuts, coarsely chopped
¼ cup hazelnuts, coarsely chopped
¼ cup pepitas (pumpkin seeds)
¼ cup sunflower seeds
1 cup unsweetened coconut flakes
1½ tsp ground cinnamon
1 tbsp flaxseeds
1 tbsp chia seeds

1. Place the ingredients in a large bowl. Toss until well combined.
2. Store in an airtight container for up to 3 weeks.

▶

TIP: If you'd like to roast the muesli, preheat the oven to 150°C fan-forced, and bake on a large lined baking tray for 8–10 minutes or until the muesli is light golden and crisp.

Protein	Fat	Net carbs	Fibre
6.4	**24.2**	**3.7**	**5.4**
grams per serve	grams per serve	grams per serve	grams per serve

Yoghurt, Nuts and Raspberries

This nutritious combo can be easily transported in a container for brekkie on the go. You can also enjoy it as an energising lunch. Note that the carb count is higher than an egg-based breakfast due to the natural sugars in the ingredients. Raspberries are one of the lowest-carb fruits because of their high water and fibre content. Adding cream to the yoghurt not only adds flavour but provides energy and helps you to feel full. If you don't like coconut cream, use regular dairy cream – or you can omit it altogether.

Serves: 1 | **Prep:** 2 minutes

150g unsweetened full-fat Greek-style yoghurt
2 tbsp coconut cream (or use double cream)
handful of mixed nuts or Dr Brukner's Oat-free Muesli
(page 166)
⅓ cup raspberries

1. Place the yoghurt and coconut cream in a serving bowl and stir to combine.
2. Top with the nuts (or muesli) and raspberries. Enjoy.

Protein	Fat	Net carbs	Fibre
15.1 grams per serve	**43.2** grams per serve	**15** grams per serve	**5.2** grams per serve

Easy Crêpes

Simple and fuss-free, our crêpes are light, grain-free and crispy. This recipe swaps plain flour for almond meal, making it a delicious low-carb alternative to regular crêpes.

Serves: 2 | **Prep:** 5 minutes | **Cook:** 15 minutes

4 free-range eggs
¼ cup full-fat milk
⅓ cup almond meal
pinch of salt
1 tbsp butter
1 tbsp unsweetened full-fat Greek-style yoghurt and
  a small handful raspberries, to serve

1. Combine the eggs and milk in a bowl and whisk for 2–3 minutes, until light and fluffy. Fold in the almond meal and salt and set aside.
2. Melt the butter in a medium-sized frying pan over medium heat.
3. Add a ladleful of the batter to the pan and swirl to create an even circle. Cook for 1–2 minutes, until the base is golden brown, then use a spatula to gently flip the crêpe and cook for another 1–2 minutes, until golden brown. Transfer to a plate and repeat with the remaining batter to make six crêpes.

▶

4. Serve the crêpes warm, topped with a generous dollop of yoghurt and a few raspberries.

Protein	Fat	Net carbs	Fibre
17.3	**25.7**	**3.3**	**1.3**
grams per serve	grams per serve	grams per serve	grams per serve

Zucchini and Feta Fritters

These veggie fritters are super easy to make and perfect for brekkie or lunch. Peas are pretty much off the menu for a low-carb diet but this fritter recipe uses a tiny amount to satisfy your cravings.

Serves: 2 | **Prep:** 10 minutes | **Cook:** 10 minutes

1 medium zucchini
½ cup Greek goat's feta, crumbled
½ spring onion, sliced
½ cup fresh or frozen peas
2 large free-range eggs, whisked
½ cup almond meal
zest of 1 lemon
salt and pepper
1 tbsp olive oil

YOGHURT DRESSING
¼ cup unsweetened full-fat Greek-style yoghurt
juice of ½ lemon
salt and pepper

1. To make the yoghurt dressing, combine the yoghurt and lemon juice in a bowl. Season with salt and pepper to taste and set aside.

2. Grate the zucchini into a bowl and add the feta, spring onion, peas and egg. Add the almond meal, lemon zest and salt and pepper to taste, and fold to combine.

3. Heat the olive oil in a large frying pan over medium heat. Shape the zucchini mixture into four equal-sized patties and pan-fry for 3–5 minutes each side, until golden and cooked through.

4. Divide the fritters between two plates, drizzle the yoghurt dressing over the top and serve.

TIP: Make the fritters the night before and simply reheat in an air-fryer or microwave for a quick brekkie or lunch.

Protein	Fat	Net carbs	Fibre
23.4 grams per serve	**16.7** grams per serve	**11.2** grams per serve	**4.5** grams per serve

Raspberry Chia Pots

Swap out the raspberries for blackberries in these chia pots, and serve with sugar-free chocolate grated over the top for a berry chocolate twist!

Serves: 6 | **Prep:** 5 minutes, plus 1 hour chilling

½ cup cashews
500g raspberries (fresh or frozen)
1 cup coconut milk
1 tsp vanilla extract
75g chia seeds

1. Place the cashews, berries, coconut milk and vanilla in a blender and blend until smooth.
2. Pour the mixture into a bowl and add the chia seeds. Stir thoroughly to make sure there are no clumps of seeds.
3. Refrigerate for 1 hour, then stir again. Portion the mixture into six individual jars and return to the fridge to thicken and set.
4. Store in the fridge for up to 5 days.

Protein	Fat	Net carbs	Fibre
4.4	**8.7**	**10.6**	**6.9**
grams per serve	grams per serve	grams per serve	grams per serve

Zucchini, Olive and Feta Bread

Breakfast is often the hardest meal to incorporate vegetables into. With this zucchini loaf you'll start your day with something delicious that, unlike store-bought pastries, won't spike blood sugar levels. This savoury bread is so flavourful – it's perfect served on its own or with a simple smear of butter.

Serves: 10 | **Prep:** 20 minutes | **Cook:** 50 minutes

200g zucchini, grated
¼ cup almond meal
1 tbsp psyllium husk
6 sprigs thyme, leaves picked, plus extra leaves for sprinkling
½ tsp salt
1 tsp baking powder
3 free-range eggs
zest of 1 lemon
¼ cup kalamata olives, pitted and chopped
100g feta, crumbled
2 tbsp pepitas (pumpkin seeds)

1. Preheat the oven to 180°C fan-forced and line a 20cm × 10cm loaf tin with baking paper.
2. Place the grated zucchini in a clean Chux or muslin square and squeeze out as much liquid as possible. Set aside.

3. In a large bowl, combine the almond meal, psyllium husk, thyme leaves, salt and baking powder. Set aside.

4. Beat the eggs in a small bowl, then add to the almond meal mixture and stir until just combined. Fold in the zucchini and lemon zest, followed by the kalamata olives and feta.

5. Spread the batter into the prepared loaf tin. Sprinkle over the pepitas and extra thyme leaves.

6. Transfer to the oven and bake for 45–50 minutes, until an inserted skewer comes out clean.

7. Leave the bread to cool in the tin for 15 minutes before turning out onto a wire rack to cool completely. Cut into 10 slices and store in the fridge for up to 3 days or in the freezer for up to 3 months.

TIPS: Freeze individual slices and pop them straight in the toaster to defrost when you need a quick brekkie.

The key to this recipe is squeezing as much liquid as possible from the grated zucchini. This will prevent the loaf from being too wet.

Protein	Fat	Net carbs	Fibre
8 grams per serve	**22** grams per serve	**8** grams per serve	**3** grams per serve

'Noatmeal' Overnight Oats

This is a great portable brekkie. Pop the ingredients in a jar the night before, then the next morning stir through and enjoy!

Serves: 2 | **Prep:** 2 minutes, plus overnight chilling

2 tbsp chia seeds
2 tbsp sesame seeds
¼ cup desiccated coconut
¾ cup coconut milk
2 tbsp unsweetened full-fat Greek-style yoghurt
½ cup mixed berries, such as blueberries and strawberries, sliced
½ cup walnuts (or your favourite nuts), roughly chopped

1. Combine the chia seeds, sesame seeds and desiccated coconut in a jar.
2. Add the coconut milk, stir to combine and place in the fridge overnight (or at least 30 minutes) for the chia seeds to swell.
3. When ready to serve, stir through the yoghurt and sprinkle over the berries and chopped walnuts.

Protein	Fat	Net carbs	Fibre
9.3 grams per serve	**39.5** grams per serve	**8.1** grams per serve	**13.3** grams per serve

Power Brekkie

Packed with healthy fats and protein, this brekkie will keep you going! Add chilli flakes for a burst of heat.

Serves: 2 | **Prep:** 5 minutes | **Cook:** 8 minutes

1 tbsp olive oil

2 free-range eggs

4 bacon rashers

1 avocado, sliced

4 slices Swiss cheese

100g rocket

1 spring onion, chopped

1. Heat the olive oil in a large frying pan over medium heat. Add the bacon on one side of the pan and cook for 3 minutes. Turn the bacon over.
2. Cook the eggs on the other side of the pan for 3 minutes or until cooked to your liking.
3. Divide the avocado, cheese, rocket, bacon and eggs between two plates. Sprinkle with chopped onions and serve.

Protein	Fat	Net carbs	Fibre
33	**46**	**4**	**4**
grams per serve	grams per serve	grams per serve	grams per serve

Scrambled Eggs with Smoked Salmon and Avocado

Scrambled eggs cooked with butter and paired with fresh sides is a fortifying meal at any time of the day. If you're feeling hungrier than usual, add another egg – or two! Keep an eye on the butter in the pan to ensure it doesn't burn.

Serves: 1 | **Prep:** 5 minutes | **Cook:** 3 minutes

2 slices smoked salmon
½ medium avocado
1 small tomato, quartered
2 large free-range eggs
salt and pepper
2 tbsp butter

1. Arrange the smoked salmon, avocado and tomato on a plate.
2. Crack the eggs into a bowl, add a pinch of salt, and whisk to combine.
3. Melt 1 tbsp of the butter in a non-stick frying pan over medium–high heat until bubbling. Add the egg, stir for 30 seconds or so, then add the remaining butter. Keep stirring, melting the butter through the egg, for a further 1–2 minutes, until scrambled to your liking (the residual heat will

▶

continue to cook the egg a little once removed from the stove).

4. Spoon the scrambled egg next to the smoked salmon, season with salt and pepper and serve.

Protein	Fat	Net carbs	Fibre
27.3 grams per serve	**48.6** grams per serve	**4.1** grams per serve	**7.3** grams per serve

Breakfast

Cheese Omelette

Eggs and cheese are kitchen staples that are often on hand, making this a go-to recipe when other protein supplies are low. Omelettes are quick to make, delicious and satisfying for any meal. Mix it up by adding your favourite veggies, herbs or smallgoods. Swap the sides out for any low-carb veg you have on hand.

Serves: 1 | **Prep:** 5 minutes | **Cook:** 5 minutes

2 large free-range eggs
salt and pepper
50g cheddar cheese, grated or sliced
1 tbsp butter
5 cherry tomatoes, halved
½ medium avocado

1. Crack the eggs into a bowl and whisk to combine. Season with salt and pepper.
2. Melt the butter in a small frying pan over medium heat. Pour in the egg and swirl the pan until the egg covers the base. Scatter the cheese on one side of the egg.
3. Reduce the heat to medium–low and cook for 3 minutes, until the egg starts to set and the cheese melts.

▶

4. Using a spatula, fold the omelette in half, transfer to a plate and serve hot with the tomato and avocado on the side.

Protein	Fat	Net carbs	Fibre
26.8	**47.8**	**1.5**	**6.6**
grams per serve	grams per serve	grams per serve	grams per serve

Three-seed Bread

An easy and tasty bread recipe that also freezes beautifully – simply cut into slices, wrap them individually and freeze for up to a month. This versatile bread can be served as a side to your meals and is great for mopping up sauces. It also makes an ideal lunch or snack on the go, paired with your favourite toppings. Slice into smaller pieces for bite-sized accompaniments to a cheese platter.

Serves: 12 | **Prep:** 10 minutes | **Cook:** 45 minutes

⅓ cup coconut flour

1 cup psyllium husk

¼ cup chia seeds

⅔ cup pepitas (pumpkin seeds)

¾ cup sunflower seeds, plus 2 tsp extra for sprinkling

1 tbsp baking powder

½ tsp salt

4 free-range eggs

75g unsalted butter, melted

1. Preheat the oven to 180°C (160°C fan-forced). Line a 20cm × 10cm loaf tin with baking paper, allowing the paper to overhang the two long sides.

▶

2. Combine the coconut flour, psyllium husk, chia seeds, pepitas, sunflower seeds, baking powder and salt in a large bowl.

3. Whisk together the eggs and 1½ cups water in a jug, then add to flour mixture and stir until well combined. Stir through the melted butter.

4. Spoon the mixture into the prepared tin, smooth the surface with the back of a spoon and sprinkle the extra sunflower seeds over the top. Transfer to the oven and bake for 40–45 minutes or until golden and a skewer inserted into the centre comes out clean.

5. Allow the bread to cool in the tin for 5 minutes, then remove from the tin using the baking paper to assist you and transfer to a wire rack to cool completely.

TIP: *Try some of our fave toppings below:*

1. *Cream cheese and cucumber*

2. *Healthy Mayonnaise (page 252), ham and sliced tomato*

3. *Vegemite and avocado (weird, but it works!)*

Protein	Fat	Net carbs	Fibre
8.4 grams per serve	**16.9** grams per serve	**3.9** grams per serve	**12.5** grams per serve

Lunch

Thai Beef Salad

A Thai beef salad is a classic dish that lets the fresh flavours speak for themselves! We've used roast beef in this recipe, which you can buy from the deli counter, but you could use finely sliced cooked steak instead. This is a great option for a quick on-the-go lunch.

Serves: 2 | **Prep:** 15 minutes

200g store-bought roast beef, roughly torn or sliced
1 Lebanese cucumber, sliced
2 tomatoes, sliced
¼ red onion, finely sliced
1 cup bean sprouts
¼ cup mint leaves, chopped
¼ cup coriander leaves, chopped
¼ cup cashews, toasted

THAI-STYLE DRESSING
juice of 1 lime
2 tbsp fish sauce
1 tbsp tamari
1 long red chilli, finely chopped
1 garlic clove, minced
¼ cup coriander, chopped
1 tbsp olive oil

▶

1. To make the Thai-style dressing, place all of the ingredients in a small bowl or jar. Whisk or shake to combine.
2. Place the beef, salad vegetables, herbs and cashews in a large bowl and pour over the dressing. Toss to combine and serve.

TIPS: If you prefer to use steak, replace the roast beef with 200g steak of your choice, cooked to your liking and sliced.

Check the ingredients of your fish sauce and tamari and opt for brands without sugar.

Protein	Fat	Net carbs	Fibre
26	**17.9**	**13.9**	**3**
grams per serve	grams per serve	grams per serve	grams per serve

Mish-Mash Hash

Instead of eggs with toast, try stir-fried veg instead! Get creative with your leftovers by using whatever vegetables you have in the fridge. If you love chilli, add some while cooking or serve with some sriracha chilli sauce on the side – just check the sugar content before you buy.

Serves: 2 | **Prep:** 5 minutes | **Cook:** 5 minutes

2 tbsp coconut oil
4 middle bacon rashers (omit if making
   a vegetarian option)
½ red onion, finely sliced
1 medium carrot, sliced into matchsticks
1 cup baby spinach leaves
4 large free-range eggs
snipped chives, to serve (optional)

1. Melt the coconut oil in a large frying pan over medium–high heat, add the bacon (if using) and cook for 1 minute. Add the onion and carrot and sauté for 3 minutes, until softened. Stir through the spinach.
2. If your pan is big enough, crack the eggs into the pan and fry them next to your veggies.

▶

Alternatively, transfer the veggies to a plate and cook the eggs separately.

3. Serve the eggs next to your veggie hash (or on top if you'd like the runny egg yolks to mix through your veggies), with a few snipped chives scattered over the top.

TIP: *Don't overcook the eggs – the runny yolks will provide an eggy sauce that is delicious with the veg. Yum!*

Protein	Fat	Net carbs	Fibre
35	**33.1**	**6.9**	**3.6**
grams per serve	grams per serve	grams per serve	grams per serve

Super Simple Salmon Omelette

Our salmon omelette is super simple to make and truly delicious! Salmon and eggs are a classic combo and loaded with healthy fats, making this recipe a great choice for a filling lunch.

Serves: 2 | **Prep:** 5 minutes | **Cook:** 6 minutes

1 tbsp butter
3 free-range eggs, whisked
salt and pepper
85g smoked salmon

1. Melt the butter in a frying pan over medium heat.
2. Season the egg with salt and pepper, then pour the mixture into the pan and swirl the egg until the pan is evenly coated.
3. Cook the egg for 3–4 minutes, until it begins to set, then cover with a lid and cook for a further 2 minutes.
4. Remove the pan from the heat, fold the omelette in half and divide between two plates.
5. Top the omelette with the salmon and serve.

▶

TIP: *If you like your omelette gooey in the centre, leave the omelette uncovered in step 3 and omit the extra cooking time; simply fold in half and serve.*

Protein	Fat	Net carbs	Fibre
34.6	**34.9**	**1.8**	**0**
grams per serve	grams per serve	grams per serve	grams per serve

Easy Ham and Veggie Wraps

Good-quality leg ham is a fantastic protein source that doesn't require cooking. Our easy wraps boast the deliciousness of a cafe lunch without the carbohydrates.

Serves: 2 | **Prep:** 10 minutes | **Cook:** 1 minute

4 silverbeet leaves, white stems removed
300g leg ham, sliced
2 tbsp Healthy Mayonnaise (page 252)
½ avocado, sliced
salt and pepper
4 pickled cucumbers, finely sliced lengthways
½ cup alfalfa sprouts

1. Bring a saucepan of water to a rolling simmer. Holding the silverbeet with tongs, quickly blanch the leaves in the water for 30 seconds, then flip and blanch the opposite ends for another 20 seconds. Transfer the leaves to paper towel or a clean tea towel and allow the water to drain, then leave to cool to room temperature. Pat any remaining moisture from the leaves.
2. To assemble the wraps, place the prepared silverbeet leaves on a chopping board and layer

▶

the ham on top. Spread the mayo over the ham and top with the avocado. Season with salt and pepper.

3. Add the sliced pickles and alfalfa sprouts and carefully roll the silverbeet leaves into wraps. You may wish to fold in the bottom to prevent the fillings from falling out.

TIPS: Want a quicker version? Skip the silverbeet leaves and use the ham itself as the wrap!

We recommend making your own mayonnaise, as store-bought versions are usually full of seed oils and added sugar. Find our recipe for Healthy Mayonnaise on page 252.

A dark, leafy green veg, silverbeet is also known as chard.

Protein	Fat	Net carbs	Fibre
32.4	**26.3**	**10.7**	**6.4**
grams per serve	grams per serve	grams per serve	grams per serve

Dr Brukner's Bacon and Avocado Salad

Dr Brukner's salad is one of the Defeat Diabetes Program faves – and for good reason! Feeling particularly hungry? Add some extra bacon or a soft-boiled egg. Feta is a great way to include salt to your diet, which can help with sugar cravings.

Serves: 4 | **Prep:** 10 minutes | **Cook:** 5 minutes

2 tbsp olive oil, plus 1 tsp extra

175g middle bacon rashers, rind removed,
   roughly chopped

2 baby cos lettuces, leaves roughly chopped

1 Lebanese cucumber, sliced

1 avocado, sliced

40g feta, crumbled

1 tbsp balsamic vinegar

1. Heat the 1 teaspoon of olive oil in a large non-stick frying pan over medium–high heat. Add the bacon and fry for 5 minutes, until crispy.
2. Combine the lettuce, cucumber, avocado, feta and bacon in a large bowl.

▶

3. Whisk the 2 tablespoons of olive oil and the balsamic vinegar in a small bowl until well combined, then pour the dressing over the salad and toss to combine. Serve.

Protein	Fat	Net carbs	Fibre
18	**29.7**	**8.3**	**3.7**
grams per serve	grams per serve	grams per serve	grams per serve

Chicken and Green Veg Soup

This recipe focuses on the natural cleansing properties of delicious fresh green veggies. Adding a variety of vegetables to your diet, especially green ones, provides your body with powerful plant compounds called polyphenols and antioxidants, which keep us healthy.

Serves: 2 | **Prep:** 10 minutes | **Cook:** 20 minutes

1 tbsp olive oil
1 leek, white part only, sliced
1 garlic clove, crushed
1 litre chicken broth
½ fennel bulb, finely sliced
½ cup sugar snap peas, sliced
1 bunch asparagus, woody ends trimmed, spears chopped
zest of 1 lemon
200g cooked chicken, shredded
1 tbsp white miso
3 cups baby spinach leaves
salt and pepper
¼ cup flat-leaf parsley leaves, chopped
30g parmesan, grated

1. Heat the olive oil in a saucepan over medium heat. Add the leek and garlic and cook for 5 minutes or until soft and collapsed.

▶

2. Pour in the chicken broth and bring to the boil. Add the fennel, sugar snap peas and asparagus, then reduce the heat to a simmer and cook for 10 minutes.

3. Add the lemon zest, chicken, miso and spinach to the pan and cook for 5 minutes, until the spinach is wilted and the chicken is heated through. Season to taste with salt and pepper.

4. Divide the soup among bowls and serve with the parsley and parmesan sprinkled over the top.

TIP: This is a versatile recipe that works with many different vegetables. It's a great way to use up anything in the crisper drawer that needs eating!

Protein	Fat	Net carbs	Fibre
54.4 grams per serve	**22.8** grams per serve	**28.6** grams per serve	**9.6** grams per serve

Mediterranean Eggs and Chorizo in a Pan

If you're looking for a lunch to impress, you're in the right spot. This Spanish-inspired dish is a breeze to make and looks too good to eat! Make sure you do, though. Not only is it totally tasty, but the perfect blend of proteins and fat will keep you powering through to dinnertime.

Serves: 2 | **Prep:** 10 minutes | **Cook:** 20 minutes

1 tbsp olive oil
2 mild chorizo sausages, sliced
400g passata
½ tsp harissa
½ cup marinated red capsicum strips in oil, drained
salt and pepper
4 free-range eggs
½ cup pitted green Spanish olives, roughly chopped
chopped flat-leaf parsley, to serve

1. Heat the olive oil in a frying pan over medium heat. Add the chorizo and cook for a few minutes until starting to brown.
2. Add the passata, harissa and capsicum strips. Bring to the boil, then reduce the heat to a simmer and gently cook for about 10 minutes, until slightly reduced. Season with salt and pepper.

▶

3. Make four small wells in the sauce and crack
   an egg into each well, then sprinkle in the olives
   and cover with a lid. Cook over medium heat for
   5 minutes or until the egg whites are firm, but the
   yolks are still runny.
4. Sprinkle with parsley and serve.

TIP: You can replace the olive oil with butter if you prefer a richer taste.

Protein	Fat	Net carbs	Fibre
25.2	**41.8**	**14.8**	**3.1**
grams per serve	grams per serve	grams per serve	grams per serve

Rainbow Frittata Slice

Our rainbow frittata slice is so simple to make yet unbelievably delicious. This recipe features three key nutrient powerhouses: spinach, mushrooms and tomatoes, which boost the immune system and keep you energised throughout the day.

Serves: 6 | **Prep:** 5 minutes | **Cook:** 35 minutes

1 tbsp olive oil
1 garlic clove, minced
2 cups button mushrooms, sliced in half
1 cup baby spinach leaves
100g Greek goat's feta, crumbled
10 cherry tomatoes, halved
8 free-range eggs
½ cup full-fat milk
salt and pepper
pinch of grated nutmeg

1. Preheat the oven to 180°C fan-forced. Grease a 24cm square baking dish.
2. Heat the olive oil in a frying pan over medium heat. Add the garlic and mushroom and sauté for about 5 minutes, until the mushroom is soft.

▶

3. Place the spinach in the bottom of the prepared dish. Top with the sautéed mushroom, crumbled feta and tomato.
4. Whisk the eggs and milk in a large bowl until combined and season with salt and pepper.
5. Pour the egg mixture over the vegetables and feta and top with the nutmeg.
6. Transfer to the oven and bake for 30 minutes or until cooked through and the top is golden brown.

___

TIPS: *Batch-cook the frittata in advance and store in an airtight container in the fridge for a quick packed lunch or brekkie on-the-go throughout the week.*

Go easy on the nutmeg as it can overpower the dish!

Protein	Fat	Net carbs	Fibre
14.7 grams per serve	**14** grams per serve	**3** grams per serve	**1.5** grams per serve

Simple Ploughman's Platter

An easy lunch or light dinner where the only cooking required is to boil an egg. These ingredients travel well and make a perfect work or school lunchbox.

Serves: 2 | **Prep:** 5 minutes | **Cook:** 7 minutes

2 free-range eggs, at room temperature
4 slices prosciutto
100g brie
handful of nuts, such as almonds, walnuts or macadamias
1 medium carrot, cut into matchsticks
6 cornichons

1. Fill a saucepan with enough cold water to cover the eggs. Bring the water to the boil, then gently and slowly lower the eggs into the water. Reduce the heat to a rolling boil and cook for 6½ minutes. Drain and run the eggs under cold water, then peel and cut in half.
2. Assemble the ingredients on a plate or pack into a lunchbox and you're done. (If you're toting this, peel the egg just before you eat.)

Protein	Fat	Net carbs	Fibre
32.7	**48.1**	**11.2**	**4.3**
grams per serve	grams per serve	grams per serve	grams per serve

Sesame Salmon Skewers

A weeknight winner that's ready in mere minutes! With the goodness of sesame and salmon, get your dose of healthy fats and pack in the protein. Don't like fish? Make these skewers with chicken, pork, beef or lamb instead.

Serves: 2 | **Prep:** 5 minutes | **Cook:** 10 minutes

¼ cup tamari
1 tsp sesame oil
1 tsp onion powder
1 tsp ground ginger
250g skinless salmon fillets, cut into 2.5cm chunks
1 zucchini, cut into 5mm thick rounds
1 tbsp sesame seeds

1. Whisk the tamari, sesame oil, onion powder and ginger in a bowl and set aside.
2. Preheat a barbecue grill on medium or a griddle pan over medium heat.
3. Alternately thread the salmon and zucchini onto four small skewers.
4. Brush the marinade over the salmon and zucchini and grill for about 8 minutes, turning frequently for even cooking, until the salmon is cooked through.

5. Remove the skewers from the heat, drizzle with the remaining marinade and sprinkle with the sesame seeds to serve.

TIPS: The skewers make a delicious and quick addition to a salad.

You will need four wooden or metal skewers for this dish. If using wooden skewers, soak them in water for 15 minutes before using, to prevent the wood charring.

Use tamari instead of soy sauce as it's gluten free, higher in protein and can contain fewer preservatives.

Protein	Fat	Net carbs	Fibre
27	**16**	**13**	**2**
grams per serve	grams per serve	grams per serve	grams per serve

15-Minute Mexican Burrito Bowl

A healthier alternative to a takeaway burrito, this recipe contains all the delicious Mexican flavours everyone loves, but with fewer carbohydrates. Paprika contains antioxidant properties, which may help reduce the risk of cancer and heart disease, improve immunity and even alleviate gas. Handy!

Serves: 2 | **Prep:** 10 minutes | **Cook:** 5 minutes

1 tomato, roughly diced

¼ red onion, finely sliced

¼ cup coriander, roughly chopped, plus extra to serve

1 tbsp olive oil

salt and pepper

3 cups cauliflower florets, grated

1 tsp paprika

½ head cos lettuce, shredded

300g cooked chicken breast (or boneless barbecued chicken), shredded

½ avocado, sliced

2 tbsp unsweetened full-fat Greek yoghurt or sour cream

1. In a small bowl, combine the tomato, red onion and coriander. Add 1 teaspoon of the olive oil and season with salt and pepper. Toss to combine and set aside.

2. Heat the remaining olive oil in a small frying pan over medium heat. Add the grated cauliflower and paprika, season with salt and pepper and cook, stirring occasionally, for 5 minutes or until golden brown.

3. Divide the cauliflower between two bowls and add the shredded lettuce, chicken and tomato mixture. Top with the avocado and Greek yoghurt, sprinkle with extra coriander and serve.

TIPS: This meal tastes great with cold or hot chicken. If you are eating straight away, you can reheat the chicken by tossing it in the pan after you've removed the cauliflower.

If you are preparing this to take to work, keep the chicken and cauliflower in one container and the remaining ingredients in another container. This way you can reheat the chicken and cauliflower in the microwave. Ping!

Protein	Fat	Net carbs	Fibre
53.6	**21.1**	**19.8**	**9.5**
grams per serve	grams per serve	grams per serve	grams per serve

Barbecue Chicken Salad

This salad is perfect for a midweek meal or when you have leftover barbecue chicken to use up. Choose chicken cuts with the skin on for extra flavour and healthy fats. Chicken also goes well with our Healthy Mayonnaise (page 252).

Serves: 2 | **Prep:** 5 minutes

1 avocado, sliced

2 cups shredded iceberg lettuce

½ red capsicum, diced

2 tbsp olive oil

70g parmesan, grated

2 tbsp pine nuts

140g skin-on barbecue chicken

1. Place the avocado, lettuce and capsicum in a bowl, drizzle with the olive oil and toss to combine.
2. Transfer the salad to a plate and top with the parmesan and pine nuts.
3. Serve the salad with the barbecue chicken on the side or shredded over the top.

Protein	Fat	Net carbs	Fibre
38.6 grams per serve	**59.8** grams per serve	**3.7** grams per serve	**8.6** grams per serve

Dukkah Fish Wraps

Spiced with dukkah, our fish wraps are a modern twist on a barbecue favourite. Our recipe uses basa fish, which, like all fish, is rich in omega-3s, low in carbs and nutrient dense. If you don't like fish, you can also make these wraps with chicken, pork, beef or lamb.

Serves: 2 | **Prep:** 10 minutes | **Cook:** 6 minutes

2 × 125g basa fillets
1 tbsp olive oil
2 tbsp dukkah seasoning
4 red cabbage leaves
½ carrot, grated
½ Lebanese cucumber, diced
1 tbsp tahini
1 lemon wedge

1. Preheat a barbecue grill on medium or a chargrill pan over medium heat.
2. Coat the basa fillets in the olive oil and sprinkle each side with the dukkah.
3. Transfer the fish to the barbecue grill or chargrill pan and cook for 2–3 minutes each side, until cooked through.
4. Remove the fish from the grill or pan and slice into bite-sized pieces.

▶

5. Fill the cabbage leaves with the fish, carrot and cucumber, drizzle with the tahini and finish with a big squeeze of lemon.

TIP: Look for Table of Plenty's pistachio dukkah in Coles or Woolies. This is a great mix with a delicate nutty flavour.

Protein	Fat	Net carbs	Fibre
35	**15.4**	**6**	**3**
grams per serve	grams per serve	grams per serve	grams per serve

Simple Grilled Lamb with Greek Salad

Explore the classic flavours of Greek cuisine with this simple lamb and salad dish. It's a cinch to make and perfect if you're short on time but looking for something fresh and delicious. This recipe works just as well with beef steak, too.

Serves: 2 | **Prep:** 15 minutes | **Cook:** 5 minutes

300g lamb backstrap
salt and pepper
2 tbsp olive oil
1 Lebanese cucumber, chopped
2 tomatoes, chopped
¼ cup pitted kalamata olives
¼ red onion, finely sliced
1 tsp dried oregano
½ cup parsley, chopped
juice of ½ lemon
100g Greek feta, crumbled

1. Season the lamb backstrap on all sides with salt and pepper, pressing the seasoning into the meat.
2. Heat 1 tablespoon of the olive oil in a frying pan over medium–high heat. Carefully add the lamb backstrap and leave to cook for 3 minutes. Turn the lamb over and cook for a further 2 minutes.

▶

Remove from the heat and let the meat rest while you prepare the salad.

3. In a large bowl, combine the cucumber, tomato, olives, onion, oregano and parsley. Pour the remaining olive oil and the lemon juice over the salad, season with salt and pepper and toss to coat.

4. Top the salad with the feta, and slice the lamb to serve.

Protein	Fat	Net carbs	Fibre
40	**44.6**	**5.9**	**3.8**
grams per serve	grams per serve	grams per serve	grams per serve

Dinner

Saucy Moroccan Lamb

This cheat's tagine is made from classic Moroccan spices and flavoursome lamb. Lamb mince is an affordable meat and a great way to increase the variety of protein in your diet. Double the recipe and freeze the leftovers for nights when you don't feel like cooking.

Serves: 4 | **Prep:** 10 minutes | **Cook:** 40 minutes

1 tbsp olive oil
1 onion, chopped
3 garlic cloves, minced
1 carrot, finely chopped
1 tbsp tomato paste
500g lamb mince
1 tsp ground ginger
2 tsp ground cumin
1 tsp ground allspice
2 tsp ground turmeric
1 tbsp sweet paprika
2 tsp ground cinnamon
400g can chopped tomatoes
1 cup beef stock
salt and pepper
4 cups baby spinach leaves

▶

½ cup pitted kalamata olives

1 cup chopped flat-leaf parsley

¼ cup slivered almonds, toasted

1. Heat the olive oil in a large heavy-based frying pan over medium heat. Add the onion, garlic and carrot, and sauté, stirring occasionally, for 10 minutes, until the onion is translucent.

2. Add the tomato paste to the pan and cook for about 2 minutes, until it starts to look separated. Add the lamb mince and cook, breaking it up with a wooden spoon, for about 5 minutes (avoid stirring the mince too much, as you want it to build up some colour).

3. Add the spices and stir for 2 minutes to coat the lamb, allowing the spices to become fragrant.

4. Pour in the tomatoes and stock, turn the heat to high and bring to the boil. Season with salt and pepper, then reduce the heat to medium and leave to simmer, partially covered with a lid, for 20 minutes.

5. Add the spinach to the lamb mixture and allow it to wilt, then stir in the olives.

6. Divide the Moroccan lamb among plates, top with the parsley and almonds, and serve.

▶

TIP: *If you have time, leave the lamb simmering for even a couple of hours longer as it helps to soften the meat. But don't worry if you are time-poor, though – it tastes just as delicious as is.*

Protein	Fat	Net carbs	Fibre
27.4	**28.6**	**14.2**	**2.9**
grams per serve	grams per serve	grams per serve	grams per serve

Prawn Pad Thai

Your favourite Thai takeaway is back on the menu, minus the carbohydrates! This easy, delicious dinner will satisfy any noodle cravings without derailing your progress.

Serves: 2 | **Prep:** 15 minutes | **Cook:** 15 minutes

400g konjac noodles (or 2 spiralised zucchini)
1 tbsp coconut oil
200g raw peeled prawns, fresh or frozen
1 red onion, sliced
2 heads bok choy, sliced
2 carrots, spiralised or finely chopped
2 tbsp cashews, chopped and toasted
¼ bunch coriander, leaves chopped

PAD THAI SAUCE
¼ cup almond butter
juice of 1 lime
2 tbsp tamari
2 tbsp fish sauce
2 garlic cloves, minced
4 spring onions, finely chopped
½ long red chilli, chopped (optional)

1. Place the konjac noodles in a large colander and allow the liquid to drain (omit this step if you're using spiralised zucchini noodles). Set aside. ▶

2. To make the sauce, combine all the ingredients in a small bowl. Set aside.
3. Heat the coconut oil in a frying pan over medium heat. Add the prawns and cook for about 5 minutes, until pink. Remove from the pan and set aside.
4. Add the onion to the pan and sauté, stirring occasionally, for 5 minutes, until softened. Pour in the sauce, reduce the heat to a low simmer and leave to cook for about 2 minutes, until fragrant and the sauce begins to caramelise.
5. Add the konjac or zucchini noodles, bok choy and carrot to the pan and toss until heated through and coated in the sauce. Add the cooked prawns and toss through the sauce.
6. Divide the pad Thai between two bowls, and serve topped with cashews and coriander.

TIPS: Konjac noodles are available in most supermarkets.

Make sure to look at the ingredients of your fish sauce, and opt for one with no sugar.

Not a prawn person? You can make this recipe with chicken too!

Protein	Fat	Net carbs	Fibre
35.7 grams per serve	**24** grams per serve	**17.8** grams per serve	**12.3** grams per serve

One-Pan Creamy Chicken and Mushroom

Our one-pan chicken and mushroom is full of healthy fats and rich enough to fill you up without the carbs. With a creamy luscious sauce and tender crispy-skinned chicken, you'll want to make this dish again and again.

Serves: 2 | **Prep:** 5 minutes | **Cook:** 30 minutes

juice of ½ lemon
1 garlic clove, minced
½ tsp chopped lemon thyme leaves
½ tsp chopped rosemary leaves
salt and pepper
4 boneless chicken thighs, skin on
1 tbsp olive oil
1 shallot, diced
125g button mushrooms, sliced
½ cup full-fat sour cream
½ tsp ground nutmeg
120g baby spinach leaves

1. Combine the lemon juice, garlic, lemon thyme and rosemary leaves in a large bowl. Season with salt and pepper and add the chicken, skin-side up, to the marinade.

▶

2. Set the chicken aside for at least 5 minutes, for the flesh to absorb the flavours of the lemon and herbs, or marinate overnight in the fridge if you have time.

3. Heat the olive oil in a frying pan over medium heat. Add the chicken, skin-side down, and brown for 5–7 minutes. Flip the chicken over and cook for another 5 minutes, then transfer to a plate and set aside.

4. Add the shallot to the same pan and cook for 2–3 minutes, until translucent. Add the mushroom and cook for a further 5 minutes.

5. Add the sour cream and nutmeg to the pan and stir to combine, then add the spinach. Return the chicken to the pan, skin-side up, and cook for another 10 minutes or until the sauce has thickened nicely and the chicken is cooked through.

Protein	Fat	Net carbs	Fibre
41	**41**	**8**	**1**
grams per serve	grams per serve	grams per serve	gram per serve

Chinese Beef and Broccoli

This is our take on the classic takeaway dish Chinese beef and broccoli, which is usually made with sugar-filled sauces. Try this dish for yourself and you'll see that it is sweet enough!

Serves: 2 | **Prep:** 15 minutes | **Cook:** 15 minutes

¼ cup tamari
2 garlic cloves, minced
1 tsp ground ginger
300g beef stir-fry strips
1 head broccoli, cut into florets
1 tbsp coconut oil
½ red onion, sliced
2 cups button mushrooms, chopped
1 spring onion, chopped

1. In a large bowl, combine the tamari, garlic and ginger. Add the beef strips and toss to coat.
2. Bring a saucepan of water to the boil over high heat. Add the broccoli, reduce the heat to a simmer and cook for 4 minutes. Drain and set aside.
3. Melt the coconut oil in a large frying pan over high heat. Toss in the onion and stir-fry for 3 minutes.

▶

4. Add the beef strips and marinade to the pan and stir-fry for 5 minutes. Add the cooked broccoli and the mushroom and stir-fry for a further 5 minutes, until the beef is cooked through.
5. Divide the stir-fry between bowls and serve with the spring onion scattered over the top.

TIP: *To save time, you can marinate the beef up to 24 hours ahead of cooking. Simply place the beef and marinade in a Tupperware container or zip-lock bag and set aside in the fridge.*

Protein	Fat	Net carbs	Fibre
50.8 grams per serve	**30.3** grams per serve	**14.7** grams per serve	**4.8** grams per serve

Cheesy Asparagus and Spinach Tart

With a light buttery low-carb pastry and a cheesy veggie filling, this dinner is just as delicious served cold for lunch the next day. Our recipe features iron-rich spinach and vitamin-rich asparagus, to give a boost of greens to your day.

Serves: 8 | **Prep:** 10 minutes | **Cook:** 45 minutes

1 tbsp olive oil

2 garlic cloves, crushed

1 bunch baby asparagus, woody ends trimmed,
   spears cut in half lengthways

2 cups baby spinach leaves

4 free-range eggs, whisked

150g mozzarella, grated

1 tsp freshly grated nutmeg

salt and pepper

ALMOND PASTRY

1 cup almond meal

¼ cup coconut flour, plus extra for dusting

1 cup finely grated parmesan

125g butter, cubed

1 free-range egg, whisked

▶

1. Preheat the oven to 180°C fan-forced.
2. To make the pastry, combine the almond meal, coconut flour and parmesan in a bowl. Add the butter and use your fingertips to rub the ingredients together to form a crumbly mixture. Add the egg and mix to form a dough.
3. Transfer the dough to a clean work surface, dusted with a little coconut flour. Carefully roll out the dough into a large 1.5cm thick rectangle and place in a rectangular 35cm × 10cm tart tin (the pastry is quite crumbly so use a rolling pin to help lift it into the tin). Prick the base with a fork.
4. Bake the pastry for 10 minutes or until golden, then remove from the oven.
5. Meanwhile, heat the olive oil in a frying pan over medium heat. Add the garlic and asparagus and cook for 3–4 minutes, until the asparagus is tender. Add the spinach and stir until wilted.
6. Tip the veggies into the tart base. Save a few asparagus spears to place on top for decoration.
7. In a large bowl, combine the egg, mozzarella and nutmeg, and season with salt and pepper.
8. Pour the egg mixture over the veggies and place the reserved asparagus spears on top.
9. Bake in the oven for about 35 minutes, until the egg is cooked through and set. Serve.

▶

TIPS: *To save time, make the pastry in advance and store in the fridge overnight.*

Leftover pastry? Don't throw it out! Roll the offcuts into balls and press down with a fork to make cheesy biscuits. Bake alongside the tart in step 4.

You can buy rectangular tart tins from Big W or Woolies.

Protein	Fat	Net carbs	Fibre
17.9	**36.9**	**6.9**	**2.7**
grams per serve	grams per serve	grams per serve	grams per serve

Silky Salmon Curry

This sweet and sour curry has a tangy sauce we know you'll love. Salmon is such a great protein source, full of omega-3. Our Defeat Diabetes expert dietitian Nicole Moore can't get enough of this dish – and neither will you, thanks to its rich, vibrant Thai-inspired flavours.

Serves: 2 | **Prep:** 10 minutes | **Cook:** 15 minutes

2 tbsp olive oil
2 tsp curry powder
2 tsp Thai red curry paste
2 garlic cloves, minced
2 tbsp tomato paste
400g skinless salmon fillet
salt and pepper
1 cup coconut milk

1. Heat the olive oil in a frying pan over medium–high heat. Add the curry powder and cook, stirring, for 1 minute, until fragrant. Add the red curry paste, garlic and tomato paste and cook for 1 minute.
2. Season the salmon with salt and pepper and add it to the pan, turning to coat in the sauce.

▶

3. Reduce the heat to medium and cook the salmon for 4 minutes, then flip and cook for a further 3 minutes. Finally, add the coconut milk and cook for a further 5 minutes, until the sauce has reduced slightly, then serve.

Protein	Fat	Net carbs	Fibre
41	**29**	**4.2**	**2.2**
grams per serve	grams per serve	grams per serve	grams per serve

Pork Schnittys with Buttery Cabbage

This low-carb version of a pub favourite will satisfy your cravings for a hearty schnitty. Packed full of protein, antioxidants and iron, this is a nourishing meal to enjoy with a mate.

Serves: 2 | **Prep:** 15 minutes | **Cook:** 20 minutes

¼ cup almond meal
¼ cup grated parmesan
¼ tsp lemon zest
¼ tsp paprika
¼ tsp salt
½ free-range egg
2 × 180g pork loin steaks
1 tbsp olive oil

BUTTERY CUMIN CABBAGE
60g unsalted butter
1 tsp cumin seeds
1 small head green cabbage, finely shredded
¼ cup chicken stock
salt and pepper

1. To make the buttery cumin cabbage, melt the butter in a large saucepan over medium heat. Add the cumin seeds and cook for 1 minute or until fragrant.

▶

Add the cabbage and stock, stir well, then reduce the heat to a simmer. Cover and cook, stirring occasionally, for 15 minutes. Season with salt and pepper, then remove from the heat and set aside.

2. Meanwhile, combine the almond meal, parmesan, lemon zest, paprika and salt in a large bowl. Lightly beat the egg in a separate large bowl.

3. Cover the pork loins with plastic wrap and, using a meat mallet or a rolling pin, pound the meat until flattened to around 5mm thick.

4. Dip the pork loins in the egg, then coat thoroughly in the almond meal mixture.

5. Heat the olive oil in a large frying pan over medium–high heat. Once it's hot, add the schnitzels and cook for 2–3 minutes each side, until golden brown and cooked through. Transfer to a plate lined with paper towel to soak up any excess oil.

6. Divide the pork schnitzels between plates and serve with the buttery cumin cabbage.

TIP: Prepare the schnittys the night before and store in the fridge overnight for a quick meal the next day.

Protein	Fat	Net carbs	Fibre
23.8	**27**	**5.6**	**2.3**
grams per serve	grams per serve	grams per serve	grams per serve

Ultimate Low-Carb Lasagne

A low-carb alternative to the classic Italian dish, our ultimate lasagne is made with zucchini in place of pasta, a slow-cooked ragu and, of course, a crusty cheese top to dive into. Mince is an affordable way to include good-quality red meat in your diet. Skip the 'lean' mince and go for the regular stuff for the silkiest meat sauce. This recipe can also be made with 1kg of beef mince, if you prefer.

Serves: 8 | **Prep:** 30 minutes | **Cook:** 3–4 hours

6 large zucchini, cut lengthways into 5mm thick slices
1 cup grated mozzarella

MEAT SAUCE
1 tbsp olive oil
100g bacon, finely chopped
1 onion, finely chopped
1 carrot, finely chopped
1 celery stalk, finely chopped
3 garlic cloves, minced
2 tbsp tomato paste
500g beef mince
500g pork mince
2½ cups passata
2 cups beef stock

▶

2 bay leaves

salt and pepper

WHITE SAUCE

1 cup ricotta

1 cup grated parmesan

1 free-range egg

1. To make the meat sauce, heat the olive oil in a large saucepan over medium heat. Add the bacon and allow to cook and caramelise for 5 minutes. Add the onion, carrot, celery and garlic and cook, stirring occasionally, for 10–15 minutes.

2. Add the tomato paste to the pan and cook for 2 minutes, then add the beef and pork mince, breaking up the chunks with the back of a wooden spoon, for about 5 minutes (avoid stirring the mince too much, as you want it to build up some colour).

3. Pour in the passata and stock and add the bay leaves. Increase the heat to high, cover with a lid and bring to the boil, then reduce the heat to low and leave to simmer, partially covered (just 'pop' the lid slightly off centre), for 2–3 hours.

4. Preheat the oven to 200°C fan-forced.

5. Place the sliced zucchini on a baking tray. Transfer to the oven and bake for 25 minutes to dry out. Set aside.

6. Prepare the white sauce by combining the ingredients in a bowl.

7. To assemble the lasagne, spread a thin layer of the meat sauce over the base of a 28cm × 18cm baking dish.

8. Layer some of the zucchini slices on top and spoon over a thick layer of meat sauce to cover. Spread a layer of the white sauce over the meat and lightly sprinkle with mozzarella. Add another layer of zucchini to cover, followed by more meat sauce, then white sauce and mozzarella. Continue until you run out of ingredients, reserving a little of the mozzarella to sprinkle over the top.

9. Cover the top with the reserved mozzarella, then transfer to the oven and bake for 40 minutes, turning the oven to the grill setting for the last 5 minutes to brown the top.

10. Remove the lasagne from the oven and rest for 10 minutes. Cut into pieces and serve.

TIPS: The lasagne can be sliced into individual portions and frozen for up to 3 months.

We use zucchini in place of pasta sheets. The key is to ensure that the zucchini has dried out, so you don't end up with a watery lasagne.

Protein	Fat	Net carbs	Fibre
46	**37.2**	**13.6**	**2.5**
grams per serve	grams per serve	grams per serve	grams per serve

Fried Salmon with Green Beans and Pumpkin

Salmon is a nutritious protein, packed with omega-3 fatty acids. We recommend keeping the skin on – it is delicious crisped up and contains the highest concentration of omega-3s. If you can't get salmon, use any fresh fish you have available locally.

Serves: 2 | **Prep:** 5 minutes | **Cook:** 30 minutes

140g pumpkin, sliced into wedges
1 tbsp coconut oil, melted
2 tbsp butter
2 × 150g skin-on salmon fillets
70g green beans, trimmed
50g feta, crumbled

1. Preheat the oven to 200°C fan-forced.
2. Line a baking tray with baking paper and add the pumpkin wedges. Drizzle with coconut oil and rub it over the pumpkin flesh. Bake for 15–20 minutes, until the pumpkin is soft.
3. Melt the butter in a large frying pan over medium heat. Add the salmon, skin-side down, and the beans and cook for 8 minutes, turning the salmon over halfway through cooking.

▶

4. Divide the salmon, beans and pumpkin between plates, scatter the crumbled feta over the vegetables and serve.

Protein	Fat	Net carbs	Fibre
49.2	**53.2**	**8.1**	**3.4**
grams per serve	grams per serve	grams per serve	grams per serve

Steak and Baby Potato

While our goal is to reduce carbs – especially potatoes! – in the Defeat Diabetes Program, we know that for those of you starting the low-carb journey the transition can be hard. That's why we've included our steak and potato recipe as an occasional treat meal for when the cravings get the better of us! Low-carb potatoes come under different brands including Spud Lite and Zerella. One small potato weighing 100g (about ½ cup's worth) contains 9 grams of carbs so it's on the higher end of the low-carb veg scale.

Serves: 2 | **Prep:** 5 minutes | **Cook:** 25 minutes

2 × 350g T-bone steaks
salt and pepper
2 small low-carb baby potatoes
½ cup broccoli florets
75g green beans, trimmed
2 tbsp butter
1 tsp tallow (beef fat) or lard (pork fat)
1 tbsp full-fat sour cream

1. Remove the steak from the fridge and season thoroughly with salt and pepper. Cover and leave to come to room temperature.

▶

2. Bring a saucepan of salted water to the boil. Add the baby potatoes and cook for 10 minutes. Add the broccoli and green beans and cook for a further 3 minutes.

3. Drain the vegetables and return them to the empty pan, then add the butter, allowing it to melt and coat the vegetables.

4. Meanwhile, heat the tallow or lard in a frying pan over medium–high heat. Add the steaks and cook for 5–6 minutes each side for medium–rare (or cook to your liking). Rest the steaks for 1 minute, then plate up with the buttery veg, including a dollop of sour cream on your potato.

TIP: Bring the steaks to room temperature about 30 minutes before cooking to ensure they cook evenly and the meat remains tender.

Protein	Fat	Net carbs	Fibre
80.2	**38.8**	**5.7**	**3.3**
grams per serve	grams per serve	grams per serve	grams per serve

Easy Sausage Tray Bake

There's no need to overcomplicate cooking. Sometimes all you want is no-fuss comfort food that looks as good as it tastes. This dish ticks all of those boxes and more – simply assemble the ingredients on one tray and bake. What could be easier?

Serves: 2 | **Prep:** 5 minutes | **Cook:** 30 minutes

200g mixed cherry tomatoes
1 medium eggplant, cut lengthways into 8 wedges
80g mini capsicums
2 garlic cloves, smashed
few sprigs thyme, rosemary and oregano
2 good-quality sausages
1 tbsp grass-fed ghee, melted
2 tsp balsamic vinegar
salt and pepper

1. Preheat the oven to 180°C fan-forced.
2. Place the tomatoes, eggplant, capsicums, garlic, herbs and sausages in a single layer on a large baking tray.
3. Drizzle with the melted ghee and balsamic vinegar, and season with salt and pepper. Toss together to coat.

▶

4. Transfer the tray to the oven and cook for 30 minutes, turning the sausages halfway through the cooking time.

5. Serve immediately.

TIPS: *We recommend buying your sausages from the butcher and having a chat about what goes into them. Sausages from the supermarket commonly have bread and other fillers, so be sure to find ones that are made with just the good stuff! Look for sausages made with 100 per cent meat to keep the carbs down.*

Olive oil can be used instead of ghee, if preferred.

Protein	Fat	Net carbs	Fibre
13.2	**20.6**	**14.9**	**10.6**
grams per serve	grams per serve	grams per serve	grams per serve

Margherita Pizza

Not only is this pizza lower in carbohydrates and sodium than regular pizza, it's high in fibre, antioxidants, vitamins and minerals, and can also aid weight control.

Serves: 1 | **Prep:** 10 minutes | **Cook:** 35 minutes

1 small head cauliflower (around 15cm diameter)
2 free-range eggs, beaten
1 tbsp dried basil
¾ cup grated mozzarella cheese
salt and pepper
olive oil, for brushing

FOR THE TOPPING
½ cup passata
200g ball buffalo mozzarella, thinly sliced
2 cups rocket

1. Preheat the oven to 190°C. Line a baking tray with baking paper.
2. Using a small sharp knife, separate the cauliflower into smaller florets. Place the florets in a food processor and blitz until the mixture has a rice-like texture (a few larger chunks are okay). You can also use a stick blender to do this – simply blitz

▶

the florets in a metal bowl in smaller batches. Alternatively, you can finely grate the cauliflower or some supermarkets now sell cauliflower rice in packs, if you prefer to skip this step.

3. Spread the cauliflower rice evenly in a thin layer on the prepared tray, then transfer to the oven and cook for 8 minutes.

4. Remove the tray from the oven and increase the oven temperature to 230°C.

5. Set the cauliflower rice aside for 5–10 minutes, until cool enough to handle.

6. Line a large bowl with a clean tea towel or Chux cloth. Tip the cooled rice into the tea towel or Chux, pull together the four corners and hold in one hand and use the other hand to squeeze out as much liquid as possible into the bowl. Open up the cloth and move the cauliflower around, then repeat the process. Squeeze really hard! You want the rice to be as dry as possible so that it bonds and crisps up as it cooks. At the end, you should be left with a cauliflower mash that's very dry.

7. Transfer the squeezed cauliflower to a large clean mixing bowl. Add the beaten egg, basil and grated mozzarella, season with salt and pepper, and mix well.

8. Line a baking tray with baking paper and brush with olive oil. Tip the cauliflower mixture onto the tray and flatten it with your hands into a pizza

▶

dough shape about 1cm thick. Transfer the tray to the oven and bake for 15–20 minutes, until golden brown.

9. Carefully flip the pizza base onto a fresh sheet of baking paper. Return the pizza base to the oven for a few minutes until the other side is golden.

10. Remove the tray from the oven and ladle the passata across the base and scatter with mozzarella slices. Return the pizza base to the oven for 7 minutes, until the cheese is melted.

11. Remove the tray from the oven and allow the pizza to cool slightly. Sprinkle with rocket, season with salt and pepper and serve immediately.

TIP: Feel free to mix up your toppings. Asparagus and parmesan is a great combo too!

Protein	Fat	Net carbs	Fibre
28.5	**21**	**8.4**	**3.5**
grams per serve	grams per serve	grams per serve	grams per serve

Learn more

Scan the QR code to watch a video tutorial on how to make the Margherita Pizza base.

Zucchini Carbonara

A nutritious, low-carb alternative to the classic Italian carbonara, our version uses spiralised zucchini, or 'zoodles'. Salting the zucchini before cooking helps remove excess moisture and prevents soggy zoodles. It is also important not to overcook them. The easiest way to make zoodles is to use a spiraliser, available at kitchenware stores. Alternatively, you can use a vegetable peeler to cut the zucchini into long strips, then use a knife to cut into thin zoodles.

Serves: 2 | **Prep:** 10 minutes | **Cook:** 10 minutes

500g zucchini, cut into zoodles

salt and pepper

2 free-range egg yolks

1 tbsp thick cream

20g grated parmesan, plus 1 tbsp extra to serve

1 tbsp olive oil

50g bacon, diced (omit if making vegetarian zoodle carbonara)

½ onion, chopped

1 garlic clove, crushed

1 tbsp finely chopped herb of choice, such as flat-leaf parsley, basil, sage or thyme

▶

1. Place the zucchini in a large colander, sprinkle with a little salt and set aside for 10 minutes. Rinse the zucchini under cold running water, then pat dry with a paper towel to remove moisture.
2. Whisk the egg yolks, cream and parmesan together in a bowl. Season with salt and pepper, and set aside.
3. Heat 2 teaspoons of the olive oil in a large frying pan over medium heat. Add the bacon and onion and cook, stirring, for 5 minutes or until the bacon is crispy (omit the bacon if you're making a vegetarian carbonara). Remove from the pan and set aside.
4. Heat the remaining olive oil in the same pan over medium heat. Add the garlic and cook, stirring, for 1 minute. Add the zucchini and cook, tossing with tongs, for 1–2 minutes, until just tender. Remove the pan from the heat.
5. Return the bacon and onion to the pan with the zucchini. Add the egg mixture and quickly toss until it coats the zucchini and creates a glossy sauce. Season with salt and pepper.
6. Divide between two bowls and scatter over the herbs and extra parmesan to serve.

Protein	Fat	Net carbs	Fibre
17.2 grams per serve	**23.4** grams per serve	**10.3** grams per serve	**3** grams per serve

Quick Chicken Tikka Masala

Make your own Indian takeaway at home with our simple chicken tikka masala. Enriched with immune-boosting ingredients, such as fresh ginger, cumin and garam masala, our spicy curry will help you stay fighting fit all year round!

Serves: 2 | **Prep:** 5 minutes | **Cook:** 25 minutes

½ tsp ground coriander
½ tsp ground cumin
½ tsp garam masala
½ tsp freshly grated nutmeg
2 tbsp olive oil
300g boneless skinless chicken thighs, diced
½ onion, sliced
1 garlic clove, minced
2 tbsp freshly grated ginger
¼ cup tomato paste
¼ cup thick cream
salt and pepper

1. Combine the coriander, cumin, garam masala and nutmeg in a small bowl and set aside.
2. Heat the olive oil in a frying pan over medium–high heat. Add the chicken and cook for 10 minutes

▶

or until golden on all sides. Remove from the pan and set aside.

3. Add the onion to the pan and fry for 2–3 minutes, until just starting to turn golden. Add the garlic and cook, stirring, for a further minute. Stir in the spice mix and cook for another minute until fragrant, then add the ginger, tomato paste and cream and stir well to combine.

4. Return the chicken to the pan and cook for a further 5–8 minutes, until the chicken is cooked through.

5. Season the curry with salt and pepper, and serve.

TIP: *Double the recipe for a batch-cook and store in an airtight container in the freezer for up to 3 months.*

Protein	Fat	Net carbs	Fibre
24.8	**21**	**4.8**	**1.4**
grams per serve	grams per serve	grams per serve	grams per serve

Low-Carb Cauliflower Fried Rice

We've added carrots to our cauliflower fried rice, but, really, you can use any low-carb vegetables you have to hand. We also love making this dish with mushrooms, cherry tomatoes and chopped green beans, but feel free to get creative and experiment!

Serves: 4 | **Prep:** 5 minutes | **Cook:** 10 minutes

2 tbsp butter, ghee, coconut oil or olive oil

340g riced cauliflower, fresh or frozen

¼ cup finely diced carrot (optional)

2 large or 4 small spring onions, sliced, white and green
parts separated

2 garlic cloves, crushed

1 large free-range egg, whisked

2 tbsp tamari (more or less, to taste)

1 tsp toasted sesame oil

1. Melt the butter, ghee or oil in a large heavy-based frying pan or wok over medium–high heat. Add the riced cauliflower and carrot (if using) to the pan and cook, stirring occasionally, for 5 minutes or until the vegetables begin to soften.
2. Stir in the white part of the spring onion and continue to cook for 2–3 minutes, until the

▶

vegetables are tender. Add the garlic and cook for 1 minute.

3. Stir the egg through the vegetables and cook, stirring frequently, for 1–2 minutes, until the egg is scrambled.

4. Stir in the tamari, green spring onion and sesame oil. Taste and adjust the seasoning, if necessary, then serve.

Protein	Fat	Net carbs	Fibre
4	**8**	**6**	**1**
grams per serve	grams per serve	grams per serve	gram per serve

Shepherd's Pie with Cauliflower Mash

Forget traditional, potato-laden shepherd's pie and try our cauli mash pie instead! It's just as satisfying but altogether lighter, making it the perfect year-round alternative. Serve with a side of crisp green salad leaves for a fresh burst of crunch.

Serves: 4 | **Prep:** 25 minutes | **Cook:** 1 hour

1 tbsp olive oil

1 onion, finely chopped

1 garlic clove, chopped

1 small carrot, finely chopped

1 celery stalk, finely chopped

1 bay leaf

450g beef mince

200g canned diced tomatoes

1 tbsp tomato paste

1 tbsp tamari

¼ cup beef stock or water

½ cup fresh or frozen peas

CAULIFLOWER MASH

300g cauliflower florets

20g butter

¼ cup thick cream

½ cup grated cheddar

salt and pepper

▶

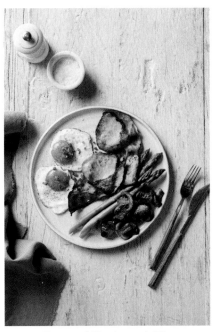

Bacon, Eggs and Veg (page 164)

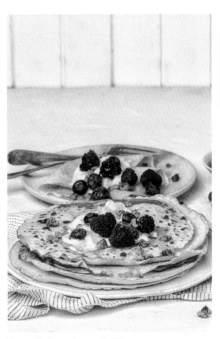

Easy Crêpes (page 169)

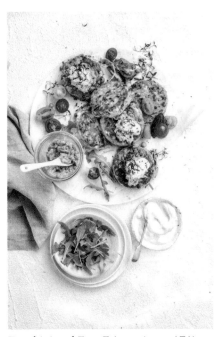

Zucchini and Feta Fritters (page 171)

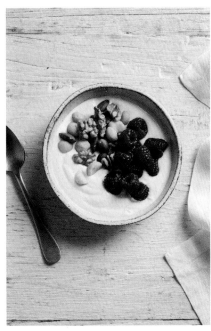

Yoghurt, Nuts and Raspberries
(page 168)

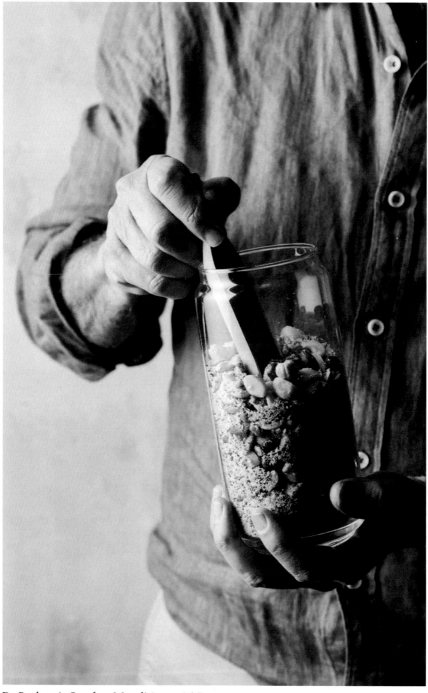

Dr Brukner's Oat-free Muesli (page 166)

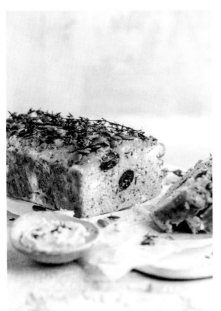

Zucchini, Olive and Feta Bread
(page 174)

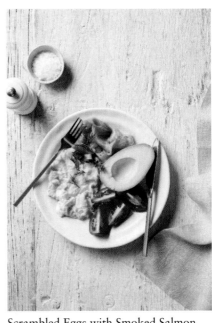

Scrambled Eggs with Smoked Salmon
and Avocado (page 178)

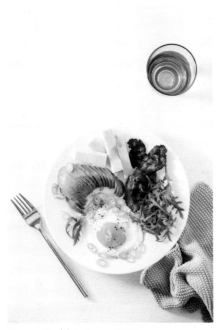

Power Brekkie (page 177)

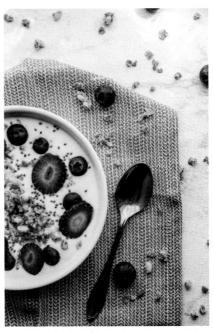

'Noatmeal' Overnight Oats (page 176)

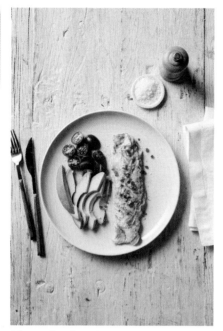

Cheese Omelette (page 180)

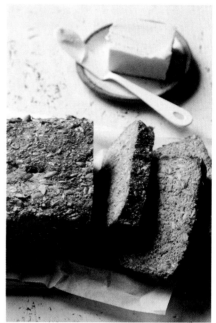

Three-seed Bread (page 182)

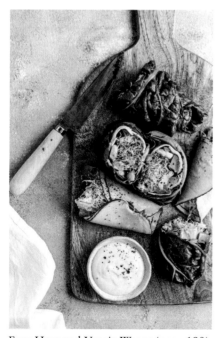

Easy Ham and Veggie Wraps (page 190)

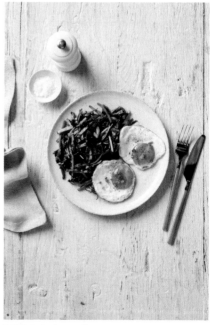

Mish Mash Hash (page 186)

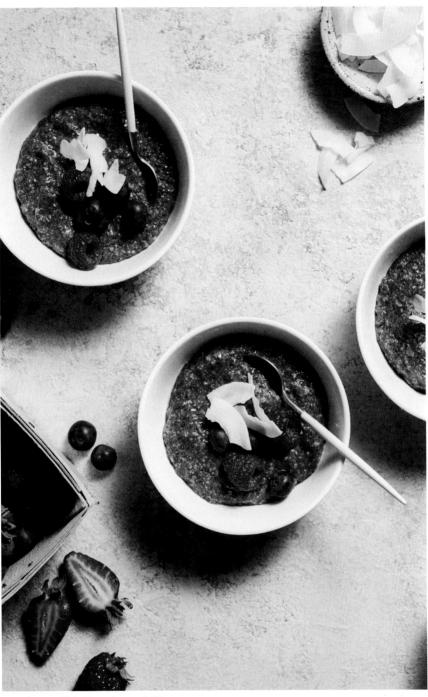

Raspberry Chia Pots (page 173)

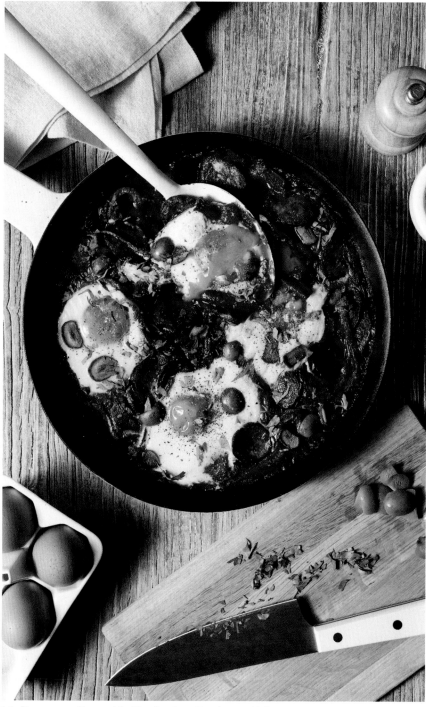

Mediterranean Eggs with Chorizo in a Pan (page 196)

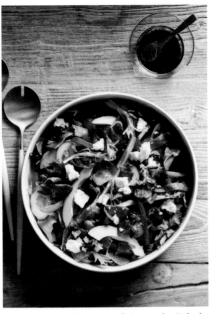

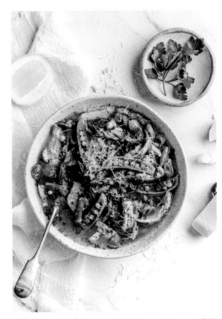

Dr Brukner's Bacon and Avocado Salad (page 192)

Chicken and Green Veg Soup (page 194)

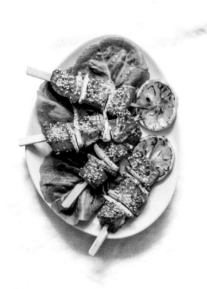

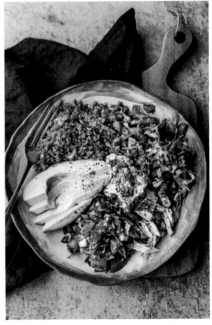

Sesame Salmon Skewers (page 201)

15-Minute Mexican Burrito Bowl (page 203)

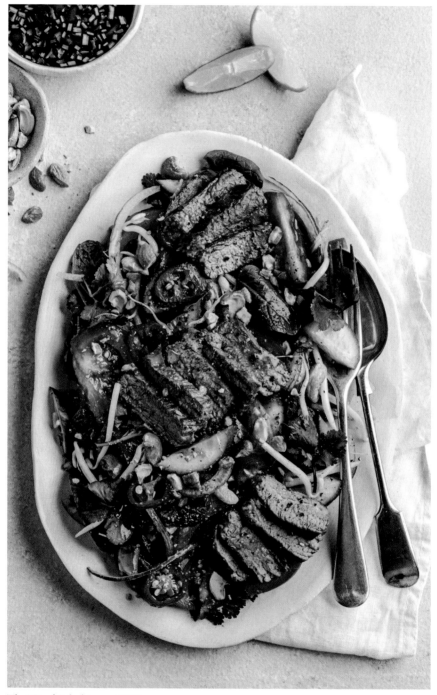

Thai Beef Salad (page 184)

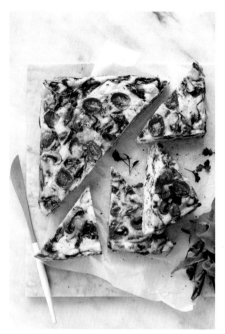

Rainbow Frittata Slice (page 198)

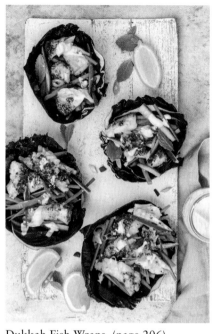

Dukkah Fish Wraps (page 206)

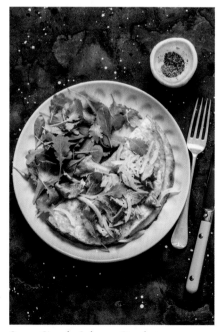

Super Simple Salmon Omelette
(page 188)

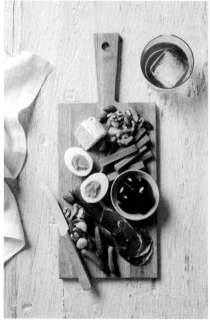

Simple Ploughman's Platter (page 200)

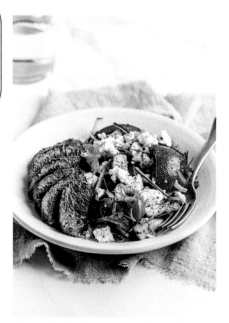

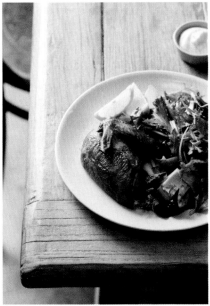

Simple Grilled Lamb and Greek Salad
(page 208)

Barbecue Chicken Salad (page 205)

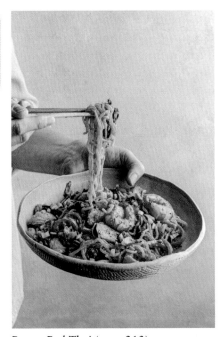

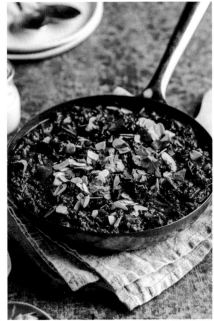

Prawn Pad Thai (page 213)

Saucy Moroccan Lamb (page 210)

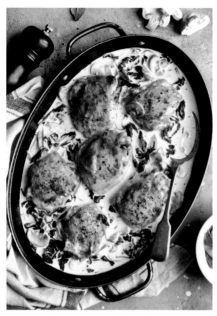

One-Pan Chicken and Mushroom
(page 215)

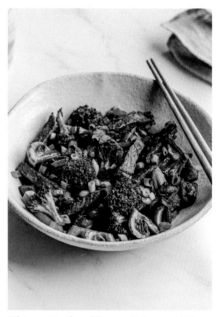

Chinese Beef and Broccoli (page 217)

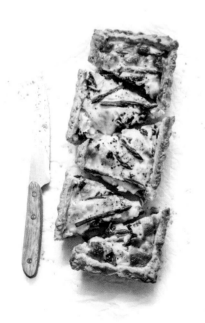

Cheesy Asparagus and Spinach Tart
(page 219)

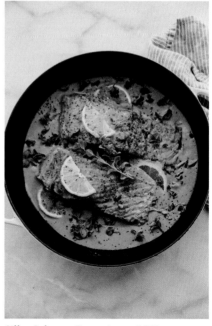

Silky Salmon Curry (page 222)

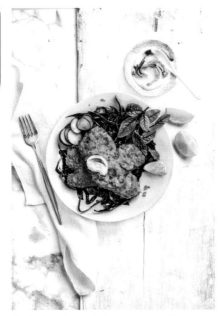

Pork Schnittys with Buttery Cabbage
(page 224)

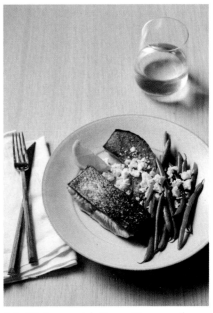

Fried Salmon with Green Beans and
Pumpkin (page 229)

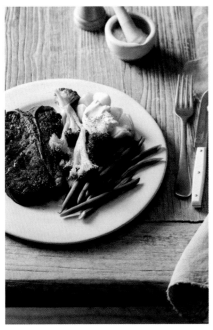

Steak and Baby Potato (page 231)

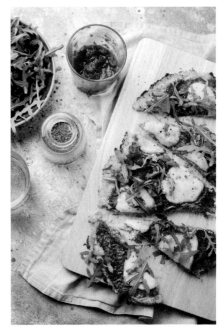

Margherita Pizza (page 235)

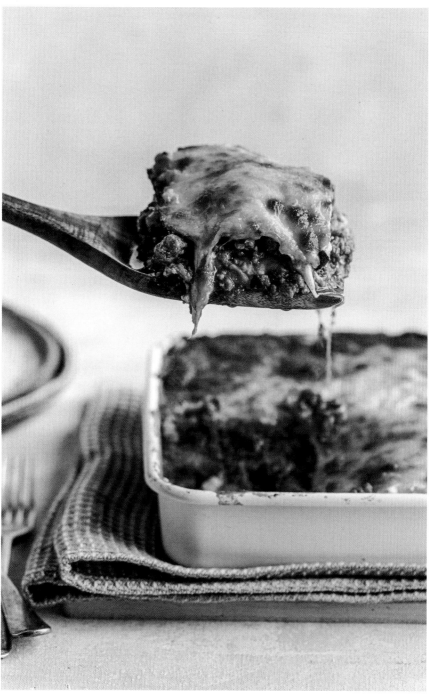

Ultimate Low-Carb Lasagne (page 226)

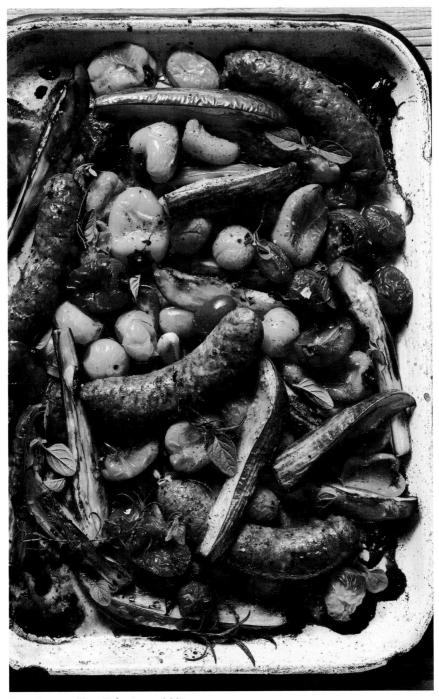

Easy Sausage Tray Bake (page 233)

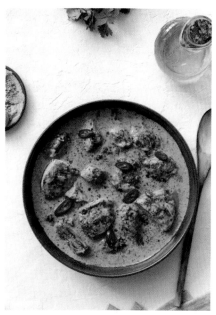

Quick Chicken Tikka Masala (page 240)

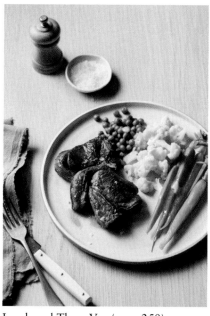

Lamb and Three Veg (page 250)

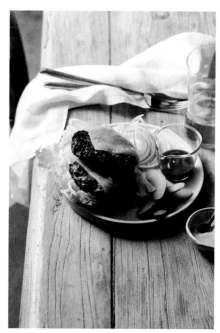

Naked Cheeseburger (page 248)

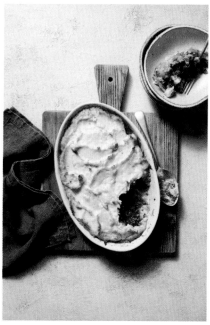

Shepherd's Pie with Cauliflower Mash (page 244)

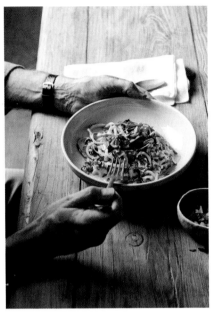

Zucchini Carbonara (page 238)

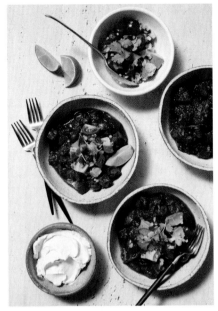

Chilli Con Carne (page 246)

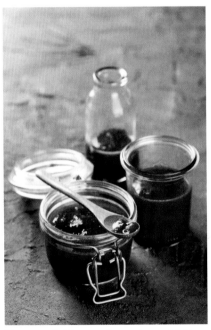

Homemade Tomato Sauce (page 254)

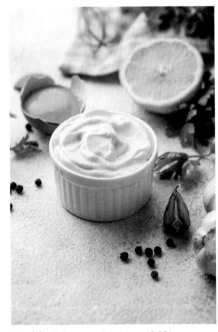

Healthy Mayonnaise (page 252)

1. Heat the olive oil in a frying pan over medium heat. Add the onion, garlic, carrot, celery and bay leaf and cook for 4–5 minutes, until softened.

2. Add the beef mince to the pan and cook, breaking up any lumps with a wooden spoon, for 5 minutes, until the meat is browned (avoid stirring the mince too much, as you want it to build up some colour).

3. Add the tomatoes, tomato paste, tamari and stock or water to the pan, then cover with a lid, reduce the heat to low and cook for 20 minutes.

4. Remove the bay leaf and stir in the peas.

5. Meanwhile, to make the cauliflower mash, steam the cauliflower florets for 5 minutes, until tender. Transfer to a blender or food processor, add the butter, cream and half the cheddar, season with salt and pepper and blend until smooth.

6. Preheat the oven to 180°C fan-forced.

7. Transfer the beef mixture to a baking dish and spoon over the cauliflower mash. Sprinkle with the remaining cheddar.

8. Bake for 30 minutes or until golden brown.

Protein	Fat	Net carbs	Fibre
30.4 grams per serve	**37** grams per serve	**11.2** grams per serve	**4.5** grams per serve

Chilli Con Carne

We've turned this traditional slow-cooked meal into a quicker version of chilli con carne. Using minced steak speeds up the process, but still gives you loads of flavour, plus you can dial it up with extra chilli.

Serves: 4 | **Prep:** 15 minutes | **Cook:** 1 hour 40 minutes

2 tbsp olive oil, plus extra if needed
1 onion, chopped
2 garlic cloves, finely chopped
1 long green chilli, deseeded and finely chopped
350g chuck steak, cut into small pieces
400g can chopped tomatoes
1 red capsicum, diced
2 tbsp full-fat sour cream

SALSA
1 ripe avocado, diced
125g cherry tomatoes, quartered
½ red onion, diced
handful of coriander leaves, plus extra to serve
juice of 1 lime
salt and pepper

1. Preheat the oven to 150°C fan forced.
2. Heat the olive oil in a heavy-based flameproof casserole dish over medium heat. Add the ▶

onion, garlic and chilli and cook for 2–3 minutes, until softened. Remove from the dish and set aside.

3. Increase the heat to medium–high. Working in batches, add the steak to the dish and cook, adding extra oil if needed, for 4–5 minutes, until the meat is browned.

4. Return the cooked vegetables to the dish and stir in the tomatoes. Cover with a lid, transfer to the oven and cook for 1 hour.

5. Remove the dish from the oven and add the capsicum and some water, a teaspoon at a time, if the mixture is looking a little dry. Return to the oven and cook for a further 30 minutes.

6. Meanwhile, make the salsa. Place the avocado in a bowl with the tomato, red onion and coriander leaves. Squeeze over the lime juice and season with salt and pepper.

7. Remove the chilli from the oven and check that the meat is tender (cook for a little longer if not). Serve the chilli con carne with the salsa and sour cream.

TIP: Use butter instead of olive oil, if you prefer, and add more avocado to the salsa for extra good fats!

Protein	Fat	Net carbs	Fibre
29	**17.8**	**10**	**5.7**
grams per serve	grams per serve	grams per serve	grams per serve

Naked Cheeseburger

Who said you had to forgo the good stuff when managing blood sugar? This naked cheeseburger contains all the burger flavours we know and love but without the carbs. For even more flavour, season the burger mince with a tablespoon of paprika, oregano or onion powder – or anything else of your choosing. Extra hungry? Make it a double patty, double cheese.

Serves: 2 | **Prep:** 10 minutes | **Cook:** 10 minutes

250g beef mince
1 free-range egg
½ tsp salt
½ tbsp butter
2 cheese slices
2 pickled cucumbers, sliced
½ tbsp low-sugar tomato sauce
½ tbsp low-sugar American mustard
¼ red onion, sliced
2 large lettuce leaves

1. Place the beef mince and eggs in a large bowl and, using your hands or a wooden spoon, mix until well combined.
2. Form the beef mixture into two burger patties.

▶

3. Melt the butter in a frying pan over medium–high heat. Add the patties and cook for 3 minutes each side or until cooked to your liking. They can also be cooked on a preheated barbecue grill.
4. Towards the end of cooking, add a slice of cheese to each burger, giving it enough time to melt over the patties.
5. Serve the burgers with the remaining ingredients on the side, or pile everything into the lettuce leaves and eat it like a hamburger.

Protein	Fat	Net carbs	Fibre
35	**34**	**5**	**2.5**
grams per serve	grams per serve	grams per serve	grams per serve

Lamb and Three Veg

Good ol' fashioned 'meat and three veg' could be accused of being uncreative – but it's a winner when it comes to simplicity and nutrition. Make this approach the cornerstone of your meals when you're lacking time or the creative juices aren't flowing.

Serves: 2 | **Prep:** 5 minutes | **Cook:** 15 minutes

2 lamb loin or mid-loin chops
salt and pepper
2 tsp olive oil
½ cup cauliflower florets, broken into 3cm pieces
4 baby carrots, sliced into 1cm thick rounds
¼ cup frozen peas
1 tbsp butter

1. Season the lamb chops with salt before cooking (half a day beforehand or longer will improve the flavour and texture of the meat, but no stress if you do it just before cooking).
2. Heat the olive oil in a frying pan over medium–high heat. Add the lamb chops and cook for 4 minutes each side or until cooked to your liking (you can also cook the chops on a preheated barbecue grill). Rest the lamb on a plate for 1–2 minutes.

▶

3. Meanwhile, pour 2–4cm of water into a saucepan with 1 teaspoon of salt and bring to the boil. Add the cauliflower and carrot and cook for 5–8 minutes, until cooked to your liking (note that smaller pieces take less time to cook). Add the peas in the final 2 minutes of cooking (or cook them separately).
4. Drain the vegetables and return them to the empty pan. Add the butter and allow it to melt through the vegetables.
5. Divide the lamb chops and buttery veg between plates and serve.

Protein	Fat	Net carbs	Fibre
40.8 grams per serve	**53** grams per serve	**9.1** grams per serve	**5.8** grams per serve

Basics

Healthy Mayonnaise

Don't get trapped into thinking mayonnaise is hard to make. Store-bought mayonnaise may contain toxic seed oils and often has added sugar, too. This versatile recipe uses light olive oil, which has a neutral flavour. It only takes a minute to make and keeps in the fridge for a week. Add a small crushed clove of garlic if you want to make aioli, or add chopped dill to partner this easy mayo with fish.

Makes: 18 serves | **Prep:** 5 minutes

1 free-range egg
1 tsp dijon mustard
1 tbsp lemon juice
pinch of salt and pepper
1⅔ cups light olive oil

1. Crack the egg into a jar or container that can fit a stick blender.
2. Add the dijon mustard, lemon juice, salt and pepper and olive oil.

▶

3. Use a stick blender to blend it up, starting with the blade at the bottom of the jar and slowing pulling it up through the mixture for 30–60 seconds, until you have a thick and glossy mayonnaise.

Basics

Protein	Fat	Net carbs	Fibre
0.4	**18.1**	**0.1**	**0**
grams per serve	grams per serve	grams per serve	grams per serve

Homemade Tomato Sauce

Love it or hate it, tomato sauce is a must-have for burgers and nuggets. Save on money (and sugar!) with our low-carb version. Store-bought sauces are loaded with hidden sugars, but our homemade recipe is sugar free.

Makes: 7 serves | **Prep:** 5 minutes | **Cook:** 10 minutes

300g ripe tomatoes, roughly chopped
½ red capsicum, seeds removed, roughly chopped
½ small onion, roughly chopped
1 garlic clove
1 tbsp butter
1 tsp stevia
1 tsp apple cider vinegar
½ tsp smoked paprika
½ tsp salt
½ tsp dijon mustard

1. Place the tomatoes, capsicum, onion and garlic in a blender and blitz until smooth.
2. Pass the mixture through a sieve into a bowl to remove the skin and seeds.
3. Melt the butter in a saucepan over medium heat, add the pureed tomatoes and cook for about 5 minutes, until reduced.

▶

4. Add the stevia, apple cider vinegar, paprika, salt and mustard to the pan and stir to combine. Cook for another 5 minutes or until the sauce thickens.
5. Remove the pan from the heat and allow the tomato sauce to cool.

TIP: You can refrigerate the tomato sauce in an airtight container for up to 2 weeks.

Protein	Fat	Net carbs	Fibre
1	**2**	**2**	**1**
gram per serve	grams per serve	grams per serve	gram per serve

16

How we can defeat diabetes

While this book gives you all the necessary tools to tackle your health issue, whether that is fully diagnosed type 2 diabetes, pre-diabetes, metabolic syndrome, or if you have a family history of type 2 diabetes or just need to lose some weight, you can gain community support through the Defeat Diabetes Program.

The Defeat Diabetes Program is based on the principle that the most effective means to control blood glucose and, in many cases, put type 2 diabetes into remission is restricting your carbohydrate intake.

The Defeat Diabetes Program is unique in that:

▶ It is Australian
▶ It is not celebrity-based, but has been created by qualified doctors and dietitians
▶ It is backed by the latest scientific evidence

The first thing we do when you subscribe to the Defeat Diabetes Program is give you a letter for your doctor, telling them what the program is about so they know exactly what changes you are making and, if necessary, can adjust your medication.

The program can be accessed online and via a mobile app. It includes:

- ▶ Thirteen video lessons
- ▶ Masterclasses, which dive into greater depth on important topics
- ▶ Articles on a wide range of subjects to improve your health
- ▶ Troubleshooting videos with my team of medical experts
- ▶ Weekly meal plans
- ▶ Hundreds of simple, affordable recipes
- ▶ Cooking demonstrations
- ▶ Exclusive live webinars
- ▶ A vibrant members' community group to share support and information

Does it work?

There is ample evidence in the scientific research literature that shows that low-carbohydrate eating is an effective means of improving blood glucose control, losing weight and putting type 2 diabetes into remission.

Web-based and app-based programs in the UK and US have also been shown to be highly effective, with remission rates around 50 per cent, significant weight loss and improvement in other health markers.

Defeat Diabetes is conducting a research trial through La Trobe University in Melbourne, examining the efficacy of the program over 12 months. In the meantime, a survey after three months of the Defeat Diabetes Program showed 63 per cent remission of type 2 diabetes and weight loss of an average 8kg.

CASE STUDY | Tina DeZen

Weight loss: 13kg in five months

HbA1c: 8.4 to 5.7 (no longer in type 2 diabetes range)

Age: 63

Summary: As a nurse with a 47-year healthcare career, Tina thought she knew how to manage her type 2 diabetes. For six years, she followed the advice of her diabetes educator and her GP, but nothing worked. After trying every 'diet' out there, and reading an overwhelming amount of information, Tina decided to give Defeat Diabetes a go – after all, she'd tried everything else!

In just five months, she has lost 13kg and seen her HbA1c go from 8.4 to 5.7.

Story: As a nurse, it's been my job to advise people on their health for so long, I thought I knew how to manage mine. I researched everything about type 2 diabetes and consulted all the right medical professionals. But nothing was working.

After going on the Defeat Diabetes Program, I immediately started to feel better. My sleep improved, I had more energy to play with my grandchildren and I finally felt like I'd found a program that worked!

The lessons were the exact education I needed.

They have shown me that you can't simply know about diabetes as a condition, you have to know what it's doing to your body. You have to understand the impact.

It has challenged all my beliefs in what I thought to be true, and I can now see the advice I was given previously is all wrong. I can see now that what I was doing before was never going to help my condition.

I also started consultations with Defeat Diabetes dietitian Nicole Moore. She helped me understand the role low-carb eating has in managing type 2 diabetes, which was a really helpful way to consolidate the education.

The best thing is that I have my hope back! A low-carb diet has completely changed my life . . . I am living proof it works.

Learn more

If you'd like to explore how you too might achieve type 2 diabetes remission through simple changes to diet, visit defeatdiabetes.com.au or scan the QR code to learn more about our members' successes.

Acknowledgements

Huge thanks to the fantastic Defeat Diabetes team, especially our wonderful CEO, Zoe Eaton, and my colleagues Dr Paul Mason and dietitian Nicole Moore. Thank you also to the many thousands in the Defeat Diabetes community who have successfully completed the program and given us great feedback, which we always appreciate. You inspire us to keep going.

Thank you also to the Pan Macmillan crew: publishing director Ingrid Ohlsson, who encouraged us to go ahead with this project, and our eagle-eyed editor Danielle Walker.

Glossary

Amino acids

Amino acids are molecules that combine to form proteins.

Body mass index (BMI)

BMI is a measure of obesity calculated by dividing your weight in kilograms by the square of your height in metres.

BMI levels and weight classifications

Weight classification	BMI level
Underweight	<18.5
Normal	18.5–24.9
Overweight	25.0–29.9
Obesity I	30.0–34.9
Obesity II	35.0–39.9
Extreme obesity III	>40.0

Continuous glucose monitor (CGM)

CGM is a medical device worn on the skin that provides continuous real-time blood glucose readings. For more on CGM, see page 28.

Diabetes

A chronic disease associated with abnormally high levels of the sugar glucose in the blood. There are a number of different types of diabetes, including type 1 diabetes, type 2 diabetes, gestational diabetes, pre-diabetes and latent auto-immune diabetes in adults (LADA). For more on the types of diabetes, see page 21.

Essential amino acids

Essential amino acids are amino acids that cannot be synthesised by humans and must be obtained from diet.

Fasting blood glucose

Fasting blood glucose is a measure of blood glucose level after an overnight fast.

Fatty liver

Non-alcoholic fatty liver disease (NAFLD) is the term for a range of conditions caused by a build-up of fat in the liver.

Fructose
Fructose, or fruit sugar, is a ketonic simple sugar found in many plants, where it is often bonded to glucose to form the disaccharide sucrose.

Glucose
Glucose is a simple sugar with the molecular formula $C_6H_{12}O_6$. Glucose is the most abundant monosaccharide, a subcategory of carbohydrates. When we eat food containing sugars or starches, the body breaks down the carbohydrates into glucose. Glucose is absorbed into the bloodstream and triggers the release of insulin from the pancreas. The body can become resistant to the effects of insulin. *See also* **Insulin resistance**.

HbA1c
The haemoglobin A1c (HbA1c) test measures the amount of blood sugar (glucose) attached to haemoglobin and shows the average blood sugar (glucose) level over the past two to three months.

HDL cholesterol
HDL cholesterol stands for high-density lipoprotein cholesterol and is sometimes referred to as 'good cholesterol'.

Insulin

Insulin is a peptide hormone produced by the beta cells of the pancreas.

Insulin resistance

Insulin resistance occurs when your cells no longer respond well to insulin and require more and more insulin to control the level of blood glucose. For more on insulin resistance, see page 24.

Intermittent fasting

Intermittent fasting refers to eating patterns that cycle between periods of eating and fasting. For more on intermittent fasting, see page 57.

Ketogenic diet (keto)

A ketogenic diet is a very low-carbohydrate diet where the body uses ketone bodies rather than glucose as its major fuel source. For more on keto, see page 68.

LDL cholesterol

LDL cholesterol stands for low-density lipoprotein cholesterol and is sometimes referred to as 'bad cholesterol'.

Metabolic syndrome

Metabolic syndrome is defined as three of five risk factors specific for cardiovascular disease – abdominal obesity, high blood pressure, impaired fasting glucose, high triglyceride levels, and low HDL cholesterol levels. For more on metabolic syndrome, see page 25.

Obesity

Obesity is excessive fat accumulation and is defined on the basis of body mass index (BMI). *See also Body mass index (BMI).*

Omega-3

Omega-3 fatty acids are a family of essential fatty acids that play important roles in your body and may provide a number of health benefits. The three most important types are ALA (alpha-linolenic acid), DHA (docosahexaenoic acid), and EPA (eicosapentaenoic acid). ALA is mainly found in plants, while DHA and EPA occur mostly in animal foods and algae. For more on polyunsaturated fatty acids, see page 83.

Omega-6

Omega-6 fatty acids are a type of polyunsaturated fat found in vegetable oils, nuts and seeds. For more on polyunsaturated fatty acids, see page 83.

Resistance training

Resistance training (also called strength training or weight training) is the use of resistance to muscular contraction to build strength, anaerobic endurance and the size of skeletal muscles.

Saturated fat

Saturated fats are saturated with hydrogen molecules and contain only single bonds between carbon molecules. They are typically solid at room temperature. Saturated fats are found in animal-based foods like beef, pork, poultry, full-fat dairy products and eggs, and tropical oils, such as coconut and palm. For more on saturated fat, see page 82.

Seed oils

Seed oil is any vegetable oil that comes from the seed of a plant. Sunflower, canola, linseed, grapeseed and sesame oils are all common seed oils. For more on seed oils, see polyunsaturated fatty acids on page 83.

Sucrose

Sucrose is the chemical name for table sugar, composed of glucose and fructose.

Time-restricted eating (TRE)
TRE is an intermittent-fasting regimen that involves a shortened time for eating within each 24-hour period. For more on time-restricted eating, see intermittent fasting on page 57.

Triglycerides
Triglycerides are a fat found in the blood formed from one molecule of glycerol and three molecules of one or more fatty acids.

Vegetable oils
See Seed oils.

Endnotes

Chapter 2: My story

14. Around that time, my colleague from South Africa…: Noakes T. My medical epiphany. The Noakes Foundation blog. Published July 20, 2015. Accessed December 12, 2022. https://thenoakesfoundation.org/news/blog/profs-words-my-medical-epiphany

14. …I bought a book, *Good Calories, Bad Calories*…: Taubes G. *Good Calories, Bad Calories*. Alfred A. Knopf; 2007.

18. In 2019, I was approached to write a book…: Brukner P. *A Fat Lot of Good*. Penguin Random House; 2018.

Chapter 3: Understanding diabetes

22. Type 2 diabetes accounts for 90 per cent...: Diabetes in Australia. Diabetes Australia. Published 2022. Accessed December 12, 2022. https://www.diabetesaustralia.com.au/about-diabetes/diabetes-in-australia

22. Gestational diabetes develops during pregnancy...: Diabetes in Australia. Diabetes Australia. Published 2022. Accessed December 12, 2022. https://www.diabetesaustralia.com.au/about-diabetes/diabetes-in-australia

29. The most readily available CGM in Australia...: FreeStyle Libre 2. FreeStyle Libre. Published 2020. Accessed December 12, 2022. http://www.freestylelibre.com.au

Chapter 4: The diabesity epidemic

35. 'The "Diabesity" epidemic (obesity and type 2 diabetes)...: Zimmet PZ. Diabetes and its drivers: the largest epidemic in human history? *Clin Diabetes Endocrinol* 2017;18(3):1.

35. In 2021 the International Diabetes Federation (IDF) released...: International Diabetes Federation. *IDF Global Atlas*. 10th ed. 2021.

36. Globally, more than one in ten adults...: International Diabetes Federation. *IDF Global Atlas*. 10th ed. 2021.

36. Approximately 6.7 million adults aged between 20–79...: International Diabetes Federation. *IDF Global Atlas*. 10th ed. 2021.

36. The overall direct cost of diabetes worldwide...: International Diabetes Federation. *IDF Global Atlas*. 10th ed. 2021.

37. One-and-a-half million Australians aged between 20–79...: International Diabetes Federation. *IDF Global Atlas*. 10th ed. 2021.

37. Two-thirds of all adult Australians are over-weight...: Overweight and obesity. aihw.gov.au. Updated July 7, 2022. Accessed December 12, 2022. aihw.gov.au/reports/australias-health/overweight-and-obesity

37. The obesity rate has increased...: Overweight and obesity. aihw.gov.au. Updated July 7, 2022. Accessed December 12, 2022. aihw.gov.au/reports/australias-health/overweight-and-obesity

37. A quarter of all Australian children and adolescents...: Overweight and obesity. aihw.gov.au. Updated July 7, 2022. Accessed December 12, 2022. aihw.gov.au/reports/australias-health/overweight-and-obesity

42. In diseases such as Parkinson's disease, Alzheimer's disease...: Phillips MCL, Deprez LM, Mortimer

GMN, et al. Randomized crossover trial of a modified ketogenic diet in Alzheimer's disease. *Alzheimers Res Ther* 2021;13(1):51; Jacka FN, O'Neil A, Opie R, et al. A randomised controlled trial of dietary improvement for adults with major depression (the 'SMILES' trial). *BMC Med* 2017;15(1):23; Phillips MCL, Murtagh DKJ, Gilbertson LJ, et al. Low-fat versus ketogenic diet in Parkinson's disease: A pilot randomized controlled trial. *Mov Disord* 2018;33(8):1306–1314; Tóth C, Dabóczi A, Howard M, et al. Crohn's disease successfully treated with the paleolithic ketogenic diet. *Int J Case Rep Images* 2016;7(9):570–578.

Chapter 5: Defeat diabetes

48. Diets of around 800 calories, often in the form of liquid shakes...: Reversing type 2 diabetes and ongoing remission. Newcastle Magnetic Resonance Centre. Published 2022. Accessed December 12, 2022. https://www.ncl.ac.uk/magres/research/diabetes/reversal/#publicinformation; Lean MEJ, Leslie WS, Barnes AC, et al. Durability of a primary care-led weight-management intervention for remission of type 2 diabetes: 2-year results of the DiRECT

open-label, cluster-randomised trial. *Lancet Diabetes Endocrinol* 2019;7(5):344–55.

50. A meta-analysis...on the effect of low-carbohydrate diets...: Goldenberg JZ, Day A, Brinkworth GD, et al. Efficacy and safety of low and very low carbohydrate diets for type 2 diabetes remission: systematic review and meta-analysis of published and unpublished randomized trial data. *BMJ* 2021;372:m4743.

50. Another systematic review of RCTs...: Nicholas AP, Soto-Mota A, Lambert H, Collins AL. Restricting carbohydrates and calories in the treatment of type 2 diabetes: a systematic review of the effectiveness of 'low-carbohydrate' interventions with differing energy levels. *J Nutr Sci* 2021;10.

52. The UK program has seen more than 400,000 people...: Saslow LR, Summers C, Aikens JE, Unwin DJ. Outcomes of a digitally delivered low-carbohydrate Type 2 diabetes self-management program: 1-year results of a single-arm longitudinal study. *JMIR Diabetes* 2018;3(3):e12.

52. In the USA, a remote care model run by Virta Health...: Hallberg SJ, McKenzie AL, Williams PT, et al. Effectiveness and safety of a novel care model for the management of Type 2 diabetes at 1 year: an open-label, non-randomized, controlled study. *Diabetes Ther* 2018;9(2):583–612.

55. In the past couple of years, it has become evident that those with type 2 diabetes…: Wong R, Hall M, Vaddavalli R, et al. Glycemic Control and Clinical Outcomes in U.S. Patients With COVID-19: Data From the National COVID Cohort Collaborative (N3C) Database. *Diabetes Care* 2022;45(5):1099–106.

55. Cardiovascular disease is the number-one killer in Australia…: Cardiovascular disease: impacts and risks. Heart Research Institute. 2022. Accessed December 12, 2022. hri.org.au/health/learn/cardiovascular-disease/cardiovascular-disease-impacts-and-risks

55. Diabetes is the most common cause of blindness…: Diabetes Australia. Changing the future: reducing the impact of the diabetes epidemic. Published November 2022. Accessed December 12, 2022. https://www.diabetesaustralia.com.au/wp-content/uploads/Diabetes-Australia-Report-2022_Change-the-Future_1.0.pdf

55. Diabetes is the most common cause of kidney failure…: Diabetes Australia. Changing the future: reducing the impact of the diabetes epidemic. Published November 2022. Accessed December 12, 2022. https://www.diabetesaustralia.com.au/wp-content/uploads/Diabetes-Australia-Report-2022_Change-the-Future_1.0.pdf

56. Diabetes is the most common cause of amputation of the lower limb.: Diabetes Australia. Changing the future: reducing the impact of the diabetes epidemic. Published November 2022. Accessed December 12, 2022. https://www. diabetesaustralia.com.au/wp-content/uploads/ Diabetes-Australia-Report-2022_Change-the-Future_1.0.pdf

57. Dr Jason Fung, co-author of *The Complete Guide to Fasting*...: Fung J, Moore J. *The Complete Guide to Fasting*. Victory Belt Publishing; 2016.

58. There is increasing evidence of the benefits of fasting for weight loss...: Saeed M, Ali M, Zehra T, et al. Intermittent fasting: A user-friendly method for type 2 diabetes mellitus. *Cureus* 2021;13(11):e19348.

Chapter 6: Restrict carbohydrates

68. The World Health Organization recommends no more than six teaspoons...: WHO calls on countries to reduce sugars intake among adults and children. World Health Organisation. Published March 4, 2015. Accessed December 12, 2022. who.int/news/item/04-03-2015-who-calls-on-countries-to-reduce-sugars-intake-among-adults-and-children

68. The average Australia consumes about 16 teaspoons...: How much sugar is too much? SugarByHalf. Published 2019. Accessed December 12, 2022. sugarbyhalf.com/how_much_sugar_is_too_much

69. The biggest contributor to added sugar intake, according to...: Australian health survey: consumption of added sugars 2011–12. Australian Bureau of Statistics. Updated 2016. Accessed December 12, 2022. abs.gov.au/ausstats/abs@.nsf/Lookup/4364.0.55.011main+features12011-12

70. Sugar content of popular soft drinks.: Bravo to 'rethink sugar drink' campaign. Sugar Shame. Published October 19, 2015. Accessed December 12, 2022. sugarshame2015.wordpress.com

73. As Professor Roy Taylor says...: Taylor R. *Banting Memorial Lecture 2012*. Reversing the twin cycles of type 2 diabetes. *Diabet Med* 2013;30(3):267–275.

Chapter 7: Does eating fat make you fat?

82. There are now numerous studies showing...: Hamley S. The effect of replacing saturated fat with mostly n-6 polyunsaturated fat on coronary heart disease: a meta-analysis of randomised controlled trials. *Nutr J* 2017;16(1):30; Astrup

A, Magkos F, Bier D, et al. Saturated fats and health: a reassessment and proposal for food-based recommendations: JACC State-of -the-Art Review. *J Am Coll Card* 2020;76:844–57; Valk R, Hammill J, Grip J. Saturated fat: villain and bogeyman in the development of cardiovascular disease? *Eur J Prev Cardiol* 2022,zwac194.

83. Research has shown that higher levels of omega-3...: Del Gobbo LC, Imamura F, Aslibekyan S, et al. Cohorts for heart and aging research in genomic epidemiology (charge) fatty acids and outcomes research consortium (force). ω-3 poly-unsaturated fatty acid biomarkers and coronary heart disease: pooling project of 19 cohort studies. *JAMA Intern Med* 2016;176(8):1155-66.

83. ...as well as having benefits for obesity and type 2 diabetes.: Menni C, Zierer J, Pallister T, et al. Omega-3 fatty acids correlate with gut microbiome diversity and production of N-carbamylglutamate in middle aged and elderly women, *Sci Rep* 2017;7:11079.

84. Their increased use as cheap cooking oils...: Simopoulos AP, DiNicolantonio JJ. The impor-tance of a balanced ω-6 to ω-3 ratio in the prevention and management of obesity. *Open Heart* 2016;3(2):e000385.

Chapter 8: How much protein?

89. The official recommended daily allowance for protein...: Diet and nutrition health advice: Protein. Dietitians Australia. Updated October 11, 2022. Accessed December 12, 2022. https://dietitiansaustralia.org.au/health-advice/protein

Chapter 9: What should I eat?

96. In recent years, some observational studies have associated the consumption...: Aykan NF. Red meat and colorectal cancer. *Oncol Rev* 2015;9(1):288.

96. The highest level of scientific evidence has failed to confirm the link...: Lescinsky H, Afshin A, Ashbaugh C, et al. Health effects associated with consumption of unprocessed red meat: a Burden of Proof study. *Nat Med* 2022;28: 2075–82; Berthy F, Brunin J, Allès B, et al. Association between adherence to the EAT-Lancet diet and risk of cancer and cardiovascular outcomes in the prospective NutriNet-Santé cohort. *Am J Clin Nutr* 2022;116(4):980–991; Sanders LM, Wilcox ML, Maki KC. Red meat consumption and risk factors for type 2 diabetes: a systematic review

and meta-analysis of randomized controlled trials. *Eur J Clin Nutr* 2022 May 5.

97. There is some evidence suggesting that grass-fed meat...: van Vliet S, Provenza FD, Kronberg SL. Health-promoting phytonutrients are higher in grass-fed meat and milk. *Front Sustain Food Syst* 2021;4:555426.

97. This is in spite of the fact that it has been known for years that the cholesterol in the food...: Fernandez ML. Dietary cholesterol provided by eggs and plasma lipoproteins in healthy populations. *Curr Opin Clin Nutr Metab Care* 2006;9(1):8–12.

98. Lactose intolerance is a common digestive problem...: Silanikove N, Leitner G, Merin U. The interrelationships between lactose intolerance and the modern dairy industry: global perspectives in evolutional and historical backgrounds. *Nutrients* 2015;7(9):7312–31.

103. Evidence shows that both a very high and a very low intake of salt...: Mente A, O'Donnell M, Rangarajan S, et al. Associations of urinary sodium excretion with cardiovascular events in individuals with and without hypertension: a pooled analysis of data from four studies. *Lancet* 2016;388(10043):465–75.

Chapter 12: What should I drink?

128. The World Health Organization suggests that the ideal amount of alcohol...: GBD 2016 Alcohol Collaborators. Alcohol use and burden for 195 countries and territories, 1990-2016: a systematic analysis for the Global Burden of Disease Study 2016. *Lancet* 2018;392(10152):1015-1035.

Chapter 13: And there's more . . .

135. There is substantial evidence that exercise can provide...: Colberg SR, Sigal RJ, Yardley JE, et al. Physical Activity/Exercise and Diabetes: A Position Statement of the American Diabetes Association. *Diabetes Care* 2016;39(11):2065–2079.

135. Regular exercise has been shown to improve blood glucose control...: Shah SZA, Karam JA, Zeb A, et al. Movement is improvement: the therapeutic effects of exercise and general physical activity on glycemic control in patients with type 2 diabetes mellitus: A systematic review and meta-analysis of randomized controlled trials. *Diabetes Ther* 2021;12,707–732.

136. The Australian Government's *Physical Activity*...: Risk factors to health. Australian Institute of Health and Welfare. Updated August 7,

2017. Accessed December 12, 2022. aihw.gov.au/reports/risk-factors/risk-factors-to-health/contents/insufficient-physical-activity

138. One study followed 1455 adults for six years...: Rafalson L, Donahue RP, Stranges S, et al. Short sleep duration is associated with the development of impaired fasting glucose: the Western New York Health Study. *Ann Epidemiol* 2010;20(12):883–9.

138. Authorities have traditionally recommended seven to nine hours a night.: Sleep explained. Sleep Health Foundation. Published 2021. Accessed December 12, 2022. betterhealth.vic.gov.au/health/conditionsandtreatments/sleep#bhc-content

Chapter 14: FAQs and mythbusters

149. It has been shown in numerous scientific studies...: Lescinsky H, Afshin A, Ashbaugh C. et al. Health effects associated with consumption of unprocessed red meat: a Burden of Proof study. *Nat Med* 2022;28: 2075–82; Berthy F, Brunin J, Allès B, et al. Association between adherence to the EAT-Lancet diet and risk of cancer and cardiovascular outcomes in the prospective NutriNet-Santé cohort. *Am J Clin Nutr* 2022;116(4):980–991.

152. Low-carb diets have not been shown to be associated with depression.: Jacka FN, O'Neil A, Opie R, et al. A randomised controlled trial of dietary improvement for adults with major depression (the 'SMILES' trial). *BMC Med* 2017;15(1):23.

Chapter 16: How can we defeat diabetes

261. Web-based and app-based programs in the UK and US...: Saslow LR, Summers C, Aikens JE, Unwin DJ. Outcomes of a digitally delivered low-carbohydrate Type 2 diabetes self-management program: 1-year results of a single-arm longitudinal study. *JMIR Diabetes* 2018;3(3):e12; Hallberg SJ, McKenzie AL, Williams PT, et al. Effectiveness and safety of a novel care model for the management of Type 2 diabetes at 1 year: an open-label, non-randomized, controlled study. *Diabetes Ther* 2018;9(2):583–612.

261. In the meantime, a survey after three months...: 63% now in remission – and that's not all our members report. Defeat Diabetes. Published 2022. Accessed December 12, 2022. defeatdiabetes.com.au/resources/our-program/63-now-in-remission-and-thats-not-all-our-members-report